FITNESS
FOR THE HANDICAPPED

FITNESS
FOR THE HANDICAPPED

An Instructional Approach

By

JAMES V. SULLIVAN, Ed.D.

Professor of Health, Physical Education and Recreation
Coordinator, Therapeutic Recreation Programs
University of Southern Maine
Portland, Maine

With a Foreword by

Julian U. Stein, Ed.D.

Professor of Physical Education
George Mason University
Fairfax, Virginia

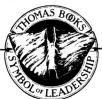

CHARLES C THOMAS • PUBLISHER
Springfield • Illinois • U.S.A.

Published and Distributed Throughout the World by

CHARLES C THOMAS • PUBLISHER

2600 South First Street

Springfield, Illinois 62717

© *1984 by* CHARLES C THOMAS • PUBLISHER

ISBN 0-398-05034-1

Library of Congress Catalog Card Number: 84-8490

With THOMAS BOOKS *careful attention is given to all details of manufacturing and design. It is the Publisher's desire to present books that are satisfactory as to their physical qualities and artistic possibilities and appropriate for their particular use.* THOMAS BOOKS *will be true to those laws of quality that assure a good name and good will.*

Printed in the United States of America
Q-R-3

Library of Congress Cataloging in Publication Data

Sullivan, James V. (James Victor)
    Fitness for the handicapped.

    Bibliography: p.
    Includes index.
    1. Physical fitness for the physically handicapped.
2. Exercise. I. Title.
GV482.7.S85   1984   613.7'088081   84-8490
ISBN 0-398-05034-1

To my wife, Ruth, and daughters, Vicki and Kaye

J. V. Sullivan

FOREWORD

FITNESS for all must be more than hollow rhetoric. **All** has got to include everyone, each citizen regardless of age, sex, race, creed, color, national origin, or **handicapping condition**. Regardless of type or severity of handicapping condition, **every** individual must have equal opportunities and access to physical fitness programs that lead to high quality, productive, and fun filled lives worth living. Programs and activities that focus on developing and maintaining appropriate levels of cardiovascular efficiency, muscular endurance and strength, flexibility, and body composition — factors emphasized throughout this publication — are crucial to persons with handicapping conditions even more so than for individuals without such conditions.

Many individuals with handicapping conditions need high levels of physical fitness components just to get through the rigors of a day of work and leisure or school and play. These needs are intensified by environments — though getting better — which are not entirely friendly or totally accessible.

Various difficulties encountered by persons with handicapping conditions have been caused, or certainly abetted, by low levels of physical and/or motor proficiency. Research results and empirical reports of poor motor proficiency and physical skill for persons with handicapping conditions can be traced and directly attributed to low levels of physical fitness — **not** inherent characteristics of handicapping conditions themselves. Basic problems have resulted from lack of expectation in what persons with handicapping conditions can attain in the physical domain, and failure to provide opportunities so that these individuals can develop physical fitness capabilities to fullest extents possible.

We live in an era in which **back to basics, excellence,** and **high quality education** are emphasized by people around the world. **Nothing** is more basic to high quality lives and the ultimate in self actualization for persons with handicapping conditions than optimum levels of physical fitness for each individual.

Too little time has been allocated and insufficient attention devoted to developing and maintaining optimum levels of physical fitness for and by persons with handicapping conditions. In many physical education and adapted physical education, recreation and therapeutic recreation programs, physical activities have been included so participants can reach other goals and objectives in the psychomotor domain — not physical fitness — or as methods to reach goals and objectives in other domains. While such efforts are to be applauded and encouraged, they cannot and must not dilute or compromise emphasis on and attention to physical fitness of and for its own values and benefits.

Framers of rules and regulations for The Education for All Handicapped Children Act (P.L. 94-142) saw this need when **development of physical and motor fitness** were identified as **first** requisites in defining physical education for implementing this legislative mandate. Many individuals with handicapping conditions have found it necessary to develop their own fitness programs since they could not find programs with appropriate fitness emphasis for themselves.

Slowly, professional personnel are recognizing the importance of and need for participation in fitness programs by persons with handicapping conditions and providing them such opportunities for participation, although to a large degree these are in special classes and segregated settings. This emphasizes another paradox in that both research and experience reveal similarities — not differences — among fitness programs for all populations, individuals with and without handicapping conditions, alike.

Review of the literature shows that physical fitness has been given limited attention in some adapted physical education texts and in some publications addressing specific handicapping conditions. **Fitness for the Handicapped** is the first publication devoted to a comprehensive treatment of physical fitness for persons with handicapping conditions. To say that such a publication has been long overdue is a gross understatement.

Jim Sullivan is to be congratulated and commended for insight and initiative in making material contained in this publication available. Jim Sullivan has presented a meld of theory and practice, physical education and special education that can be an effective resource for all involved in fitness programs in which persons with handicapping conditions take part — teachers, leaders, coaches, trainers, administrators, participants themselves.

Although emphasis of the publication is upon the **whats** and **hows** of fitness programs and activities, rationale for each of the general types of programs and specific activities is documented with important but often overlooked **whys**. Jim Sullivan draws from and integrates basics from exercise physiology, motor learning, adapted physical education, education and special education for an individualized and personalized emphasis in his practical and instructional approach.

Principles and guidelines are sprinkled liberally throughout the publication to add to ease of practical applications in either integrated or special settings. The reader is given basics for planning, organizing, administering, and evaluating fitness programs for persons with handicapping conditions. Ways to establish goals and objectives, translate assessment results into individualized exercise programs, apply general and specific instructional methods and techniques, and accommodate participants in various types of fitness programs and activities add to the practicality of this publication. Accommodation is the underlying thread throughout this publication.

With good judgment and common sense, professional personnel competent in the basics of sound high quality fitness programs can, while working hand-in-hand with participants possessing handicapping conditions, make these simple and easily accomplished accommodations. Such a process makes equal opportunities in these programs realities for **every** person with a handicapping condition, regardless of its type or severity.

Because of Jim Sullivan's dedication to a cause and commitment to equality of opportunity, many more persons with handicapping conditions will attain and maintain high quality lives in which each individual lives as long as he/she wants, and wants to as long as he/she lives.

Julian U. Stein
Professor in Physical Education
George Mason University
Fairfax, Virginia

PREFACE

RESEARCH confirms the fact that millions of people all over the world are now participating in various types of physical fitness activities. Additionally, the fitness mania has not only made people more aware of their personal health and physical well-being than formerly, but has also created a social and economic boom as well. It is a sad, but true, commentary that the fitness movement is focused primarily on the regular population, while the handicapped are receiving very little attention, if any. Professional personnel working with the disabled should be most concerned about this segment of the population's holistic health, with an emphasis on physical fitness.

The handicapped have basically the same needs and desires as the non-handicapped. One basic goal is to improve their capacity to function physically as effectively as possible within their limitations. Why, then, are the disabled not given more opportunity to take part in various types of fitness programs and activities? The most common answer is lack of money, facilities, and trained personnel.

This answer isn't acceptable nor is it justifiable. If money, facilities, and trained fitness personnel are available to the non-handicapped, they should be available to the handicapped. Equality, in so far as possible, should exist between these two populations in fitness programs. Physical fitness programs and activities for the disabled are long overdue. The world in which we live must be made a place where all people are given equal opportunities to grow and develop to their fullest potential. Changes in lifestyles to bring about improvements in physical fitness levels should be of major concern to both the regular and the handicapped populations.

The "Rehabilitation Act of 1973, Section 504" guarantees civil and personal rights of handicapped persons in all programs for which sponsoring groups receive federal funds. Public Law 94-142, "Education for All Handicapped Children Act of 1975," stipulates that handicapped children ages 3 through 21 must be guaranteed a free, appropriate, public education. In addition to these two federal laws, most states now have laws which guarantee the availability of a free, appropriate, public education to all handicapped children.

Both the federal and the state laws have helped to change the attitude of society toward the disabled. Yet, the battle is far from over. There are several problems confronting the handicapped that must be solved: education, housing, transportation, access to public buildings, accessible sidewalks, and fitness programs designed to meet their functional capacities. These physical fitness programs must begin to be implemented in both public and private schools, recreation centers, private health and fitness centers, hospitals, nursing homes, intermediate care facilities, and in institutions. The fitness movement is here; we must not overlook the fitness of the disabled population.

The strong belief I have that **all people** should be given equal opportunity to participate in fitness programs and activities prompted me to write this book. We must look at an individual's ability, not at his/her disability. We need to be offering fitness programs in various types of settings to the handicapped. Professionals who work with the disabled need to make a personal commitment to providing fitness opportunities to individuals who have various types of handicapping conditions. And yet, no one claims this task will be easy. It will take a lot of work and dedication on the part of all fitness professionals. But the benefits gained by participants in a fitness program specifically designed for the handicapped will more than reward the professionals for their commitment.

For many fitness personnel the idea of offering physical fitness programs and activities to the disabled seems unrealistic. Granted, there is a body of knowledge that must be learned. But the task of acquiring this knowledge is not out of reach of the professional. Learning is a life-long process; if the professional has determination and a sincere desire to learn about physical fitness for the handicapped, the task becomes easier than anticipated and more enjoyable.

A need exists to provide a book for professional preparation, both in-service and pre-service. As a result, this book is written from a practical and functional viewpoint for regular and adapted physical educators, special educators, health educators, resource center educators, therapeutic recreators, physical therapists, athletic trainers, athletic coaches, sports medicine personnel, and others working in hospitals, institutions, clinics, nursing homes, and private health and fitness centers.

This book is organized into two parts. Part I, "FOUNDATIONS OF FITNESS FOR THE HANDICAPPED," includes an introduction, learning about physical activity, and understanding the functional capabilities of the handicapped. Part II, "ORGANIZATION AND ADMINISTRATION OF FITNESS PROGRAMS FOR THE HANDICAPPED," provides information on establishing fitness goals and objectives, planning and organizing fitness classes and programs, assessing participants for program placement, instructing the handicapped, and knowing about fitness programs and adaptations.

Handicapped individuals, like their non-handicapped counterparts, have much leisure time on their hands and need to spend these leisure hours in a productive way. These leisure hours can easily be converted into time spent in participating in physical activities. Thus, parents, family members, and volunteers will find that this book provides information on physical fitness programs and activities and ways in which to teach them to the handicapped.

I should like to recognize the contributions of Robert W. Scarlata, M.D., Clinical Director, Pineland Hospital and Training Center; Albert Anderson, Ph.D., Psychology, University of Southern Maine; Lawrence E. Braziel, Director of Management Information Systems, University of Southern Maine; and Len Jordan, Coordinator of Cardiac Rehabilitation and Pulmonary Exercise Programs, University of Southern Maine. I should also like to thank Jenny Reed for a fine job in typing the manuscript.

James V. Sullivan

CONTENTS

FITNESS
FOR THE HANDICAPPED

Part I

FOUNDATIONS OF FITNESS
FOR THE HANDICAPPED

Chapter I

INTRODUCTION
FITNESS: STATE OF THE ART

WHERE ARE WE NOW?

FITNESS is fast becoming a social phenomenon, or a state of being, in the United States and throughout the civilized world. Yet, for all this growth and its benefits to tens of millions, the fitness trend has had relatively little impact on the handicapped.* The question frequently asked is, "Why hasn't more progress been made with respect to fitness for the handicapped?" The answer is simple: Knowledge, personnel, facilities, equipment, money, and research are lacking. But the disabled population should not despair and give up, for there is a ray of light beyond the horizon. Educators, therapists, nurses, exercise specialists, and physiatrists are beginning to realize that physical fitness is just as beneficial to the handicapped as it is to the regular population.

A review of the literature reveals that a national survey has never been conducted to determine the status of fitness programs and activities for the physically and mentally handicapped. Adapted physical education and recreation, sports, and rehabilitation programs for the handicapped are being offfered through Special Olympics, special, private and mainstreamed schools, agencies, institutions, recreation departments, and hospitals. Currently, however, what percentage of time is devoted to teaching physical fitness to the

---

*In this text, the terms "handicapped" or "disabled" are used interchangeably.

handicapped and which programs, if any, are specifically fitness-oriented are unknown. The literature indicates that outside of hospital rehabilitation departments, minimal fitness offerings are available. Until such time as a survey is conducted and the data analyzed, one can only speculate about the type, amount, and focus of physical fitness programs and activities available to the disabled population. Short-term and long-term studies* which have been conducted both in the United States and abroad have dealt with various types of fitness activities for specific types of handicapping conditions. Discussed herein are the types of handicaps which receive the most attention in terms of physical fitness, physical training, physical conditioning and/or motor functioning. The mentally retarded appear at the top, followed by the blind, the asthmatics, the cerebral palsied, the deaf, the amputees, and the spinal-cord injured. The research completed on the above handicapping conditions concluded very clearly that appropriate fitness programs and activities designed to meet the functioning levels of handicapped individuals, conducted over a period of time, will improve cardiovascular endurance, muscular strength and endurance, flexibility, or a combination of these, depending upon intensity, duration, frequency, and type of activity performed.

HOW DID WE GET HERE?

It is obvious that physical fitness per se was not known during prehistoric times, but early man needed to hunt, fish, and engage in combat in order to survive. Thus, he developed strength and endurance because of these survival skills; and, therefore, it can be said that physical fitness was practiced by primitive man, although not voluntarily.

The Chinese were one of the first people to develop far beyond primitive people and to establish one of the earliest centers of civilization. Historical and archeological records reveal that therapeutic exercise was practiced in ancient China and also in other old civilizations. Licht tells us that Cong Fou was a series of ritualistic positions

---

*Refer to the bibliography for specific titles.

and motions prescribed by Taoist priests for relief of pain and other symptoms . . . and consisted of body positioning and breathing routines.[1]

Later, in about 1000 AD, the Chinese also developed a system of exercises called T'ai Chi Chuan. This system can lead to the art of self-defense and requires inner control of the mind and body, alertness and concentration, and specific exercise structures. There are over 100 structured positions and variations in which two principles, softness and circular movements, apply. The five essential qualities are slowness, lightness, clarity, balance, and calmness.[2]

Although China and other Oriental civilizations established and practiced therapeutic exercise, ancient Greece is recognized in contemporary times as the birthplace of the philosophical concept of a sound mind and a sound body. Herodicus, 480 BC, was the first Greek to write about a system of exercises that used corrective therapy to help cure bodily weaknesses. One of his students, Hippocrates, 460 BC, a famous Greek physician, wrote many books on the value and benefits derived from exercise and included walking at a fast pace as a method of reducing obesity. In his book entitled **On Articulations**, Hippocrates demonstrated his deep insight into the relationship between motion and muscle. In addition, the Greek philosophers, Socrates, Aristotle, and Plato, recommended medical gymnastics to their citizens as the best form of exercise.[3]

With the downfall of Greek civilization, political power shifted to the Macedonians and then to the Romans. Because the latter used Greek culture and knowledge, they succeeded in making valuable contributions in various parts of the world.

Galen, 130 AD, was a physician who was born in Greece but lived in the Roman Empire. He acquired a vast knowledge about the musculo-skeletal system. In his book, **On Hygiene**, Galen suggested specific exercises for various parts of the body and further classified these into three groups: exercises for muscle tone, quick exercises,

---

[1]Sidney Licht, *Therapeutic Exercise*, 2nd ed. (Baltimore, Maryland: Waverly Press, Inc., 1969), p. 426.
[2]Sophia Delza, *Body and Mind in Harmony* (New York: David McKay, Co., Inc., 1961).
[3]Licht, *op. cit.*, p. 428.

and violent exercises.[4] He also classified exercises "according to their vigor, duration, frequency, use of apparatus, and the part of the body involved."[5]

One of the most famous Romans to follow Galen was Aurelianus, who lived toward the end of the fifth century. He had some very modern concepts on physical treatment, including hydrogymnastics and the use of pulleys and weights for kinesitherapy. Aurelianus, in the first section of his second book entitled, **On Chronic Diseases**, not only discusses the treatment for paralysis of different body parts but also describes a series of exercises that can be performed by using devices which develop muscle strength and tone.[6]

Just as the Greek Empire collapsed, so did the Roman Empire. The Christian philosophy focused on the soul and renounced body strength and beauty. Until the ninth century only lords and knights performed exercises, and even they did very little.

The Arabians, through Syrian and Hebrew translations, kept Greek and Roman medicine alive. Rhazes, an Arabian physician, wrote a book on hygiene in which he expressed the value of both exercise and cleanliness of the home. Avicenna wrote that if men exercised their bodies at appropriate times, they would need neither medicines nor physicians.[7]

Judaeus wrote, in the tenth century, that idleness is extremely harmful to the regulation of health. Actuarius, in the thirteenth century, prescribed diet and exercises as cures for diseases, especially mental diseases. Catalan, at the beginning of the fourteenth century expressed the need for convenient medicines, exercise, and happiness.[8]

The Renaissance era introduced an interest in worldly matters such as earthly success as opposed to other worldly concerns. This was the period that captivated the minds of Italy and advanced an aesthetic attitude. It was a time which took a modern view toward the body and physical activity.

---

[4]D. B. Van Dalen, E. D. Mitchell, and B. L. Bennett, *A World History of Physical Education* (Englewood Cliffs, New Jersey: Prentice-Hall, Inc., 1953), p. 93.
[5]Licht, *op. cit.*, p.431.
[6]*Ibid.*, pp. 432-433.
[7]*Ibid.*, p. 434.
[8]*Ibid.*, p. 435.

Vergerio (1349-1428) reintroduced physical education within the educational program. Because of his influence Feltra, a physician turned educator, started the Mantua School in 1423 to offer young noblemen both a mental and a physical education.[9]

With the invention of the printing press, intellectual activity flourished. Books now appeared which stressed the hygienic value of exercise. Fuchs, a professor and physician, wrote a book entitled **Institutiones Medicae,** which contained a resume on the art of exercise. Mendez wrote **Libro del Exercicio,** which was the first printed book on exercise authored by a physician and dealt mainly with hygiene. Mercurealis, a professor at the University of Padua, wrote the first important book in modern times on therapeutic exercise, a book which was reprinted five times. He established the following seven principles of medical gymnastics:

1. Each exercise should preserve the existing healthy state.
2. Exercise should not disturb the harmony among the principal humors.
3. Exercises should be suited to each part of the body.
4. All healthy people should take exercise regularly.
5. Sick people shouldn't be given exercises which might exacerbate conditions.
6. Special exercises should be prepared for convalescent patients on an individual basis.
7. Persons who lead a sedentary life urgently need exercise.[10]

During the next two centuries, several notable scholars wrote on the subjects of exercise, hygiene and treatment. In the 17th century, a treatise on hygiene was written by Duchesne, a physician to Henry IV, in which he stated, "Exercise is a salutory thing which guarantees the human body from many infirmities and diseases to which idleness and rest render it subject . . . it renders the body agile, strengthens the nerves and joints.[11]

Sanctorius authored a book on exercise and rest in which he stated, "Moderate exercise gives the body lightness and vigor; it cleanses the muscles and ligaments of their waste products and pre-

---

[9]*Ibid.*
[10]*Ibid.*, pp. 437-438.
[11]*Ibid.*, p. 438.

pares the matter for dissipation throughout the sweat . . ."[12] He also advocated both indoor and outdoor exercises.

Luther stressed the value of exercise and advocated gymnastics for a strong, robust, healthy body. He believed that exercise can keep young people from "idleness, debauchery and drink."[13]

In the eighteenth century, Hoffman (1660-1742), a physician, did most to establish the importance of exercise in hygiene and medical treatment. In his book **Dissertationes Physico-Medicae,** he classified occupational movements (cutting wood, threshing wheat, fishing) as exercise.[14]

Andry (1658-1742) renounced the priesthood to study medicine and to follow Hoffman. He related exercise to the musculo-skeletal system. One of his greatest contributions came from his book entitled **L'Orthopedie,** published in 1741, in which he gave a set of rules for correcting postural deformities.[15]

The last part of the eighteenth century saw changes in human thought and action. Tissot (1747-1826), a medical doctor, produced work on therapeutic exercise, but its full importance was not recognized for some years to come. He insisted that knowledge of anatomy was essential before one could prescribe orthopedic exercises. He is credited with the analyzation of motion associated with manual and craft activities. Tissot established the principles for occupational therapy and, in addition, prescribed the use of recreational therapy and adapted sports. His book, entitled **Gymnastique Medicinale et Chirurgicale** was translated into German, Italian, Swedish and Norwegian.[16]

The nineteenth century saw advances in medicine and education and a rapid growth in the gymnastic movement, the latter credited to Ling (1776-1830). He advocated exercise for physical and moral perfection and set down certain laws related to variation of resistance, as used in medical gymnastics. He is also credited with the introduction of dosage, counting, and detailed directions in exercise and believed in exercise for all.[17]

---

[12]*Ibid.*

[13]*Ibid.*

[14]*Ibid.*, p. 440.

[15]*Ibid.*, pp. 441-442.

[16]*Ibid.*, p.443.

[17]*Ibid.*, pp. 447-448.

Zander was born in Stockholm, Sweden, in 1835. In 1857, while conducting gymnastic exercises at a girls' boarding school, he decided to analyze the Ling system of exercise. He concluded that the relationship of only one patient performing exercises supervised by a gymnast was not economically feasible. Thus, he recommended levers, wheels, and weights to provide both assistance and resistance. The gymnast now would be needed only at the beginning of the patient's program for occasional supervision. Before he died, Zander had developed 71 different types of apparatus and devices for active, assertive and resistive exercise, as well as for massage.[18]

Stokes, an Irishman, regulated exercises and planned walks for heart disease patients as early as 1854. Mitchell, in 1874, proposed rest treatment for his cardiac patients, which he soon changed to include graduated exercise and massage.[19]

In the early part of the twentieth century, Sargent, an American physician, made major contributions by designing exercise apparatus and devices used to develop muscle strength.[20] World War I brought attention to the fact that there must be a new attitude and concern toward exercise. Because of the many young people who were found unfit for service, more opportunities needed to be provided for exercise and physical activity.

Following World War II, the attitude and concern for exercise and fitness expanded even further. In 1944, Delorme, an Alabama physician, devised a method of weight training called "Progressive Resistance Exercise," which is designed to develop muscle strength. His method of weight training is also used as a technique in rehabilitation.[21]

The fitness movement, born in the seventies, has yet to reach its peak. There are literally millions of people all over the world who are participating in some type of fitness program, physical recreation program, or sports program. Unfortunately, the same cannot be said for the handicapped.

A group of professionals and the AAHPERD, in cooperation with the Joseph P. Kennedy, Jr., Foundation, have made valuable

[18]*Ibid.*, pp. 451-452.
[19]*Ibid.*, pp. 453-454.
[20]*Ibid.*, p.454.
[21]*Ibid.*, p.464.

contributions to physical and motor fitness. They have developed the following assessment instruments designed specifically for the handicapped: "Physical Fitness Test for the Mentally Retarded," developed by Haden in 1964; "Physical Fitness in Relation to Intelligence Quotient, Social Distance, and Physique of Intermediate School Mentally Retarded Boys," a dissertation by Stein, completed in 1966; "Special Fitness Test for the Mentally Retarded Manual," (Educable Mentally Retarded), published by AAHPER and the Kennedy Foundation in 1968.

In addition, Fait, in 1972, published a "Physical Fitness Test Battery for Mentally Retarded Children." Buell, in 1973, published his "Adaptation of the 1965 AAHPER Youth Fitness Test for the Blind and Partially Seeing." AAHPER, in 1975, revised their "Youth Fitness Test Manual." Johnson and Londeree developed, and in 1976 the AAHPER published, the "Motor Fitness Test Manual for the Moderately Mentally Retarded." Vodola conducted, in 1978, **Project Active,** and published a "Motor Ability and Physical Fitness Test for the Normal, Mentally Retarded Learning Disabled, and Emotional Disturbed," and included norms.

AAHPERD, in 1980, published a "Health Related Physical Fitness Test Manual." (Items can be adapted for use with the handicapped.) Winnick and Short conducted **Project Unique** and published, in 1982, "The Physical Fitness Test for Sensory and Orthopedically Impaired Youth," and included norms.

The eighties will perhaps see the trend of testing and/or training paraplegics in cardiovascular endurance on wheelchair ergometers. This piece of apparatus may soon come to replace arm ergometers. Although testing results on both are accurate, wheelchair ergometers provide natural hand and arm movements similar to those used for daily mobility.

FITNESS: DEFINITIONS AND TYPES FROM A PRACTICAL AND FUNCTIONAL VIEWPOINT

We are living in an era in which a great deal of attention is given to total fitness or holistic health. This totalitarian concept has resulted in a nebulous approach to total fitness, particularly as it relates to the handicapped. The time has arrived that they, too, should be given opportunities to grow and develop within their functioning capabilities. Thus, the following types of fitness are briefly explained in hopes that each professional who works with the disabled will begin to realize that this segment of the population is human and needs help in a variety of ways. There are various types of fitness:

Emotional fitness is one's ability, either potential or actual, to express feelings in a manner acceptable to himself/herself and to society. Emotional fitness is a reflection of mental fitness. The healthier one's thoughts of life are, the healthier the expression of one's emotions will be.

Mental fitness is a state of harmony between reality and the acceptance of the self in whatever condition one finds himself/herself, whether physical or otherwise.

Physical fitness is one's ability, either potential or actual, to develop and maintain strength and stamina sufficient for daily living and the enjoyment of leisure. Five components of physical fitness are muscular strength, muscular endurance, cardiovascular endurance, flexibility, and body fat composition.

Social fitness is the ability, either potential or actual, to behave and interact in a socially acceptable manner, the capacity to take part in daily personal interactions appropriately for personal enjoyment and fulfillment in opportunities of giving and receiving.

Spiritual fitness is a sense of contentment with oneself and his/her relationship to God, a security in the belief that God has control over, and a purpose in, the events and conditions of one's life. A belief in being loved and accepted by one's creator may encourage or result in the love and acceptance of oneself.

KINDS OF EXERCISE PROGRAMS AND TRAINING SYSTEMS

Seven kinds of exercises and three kinds of training systems are in existence and are identified below. A logical sequence of any one of these kinds of exercises, or any combination, performed over a period of time, would comprise a program. The selection of any particular type of program, however, is an individual matter based on goals. Before any program selection can be made, two important considerations must be taken into account: the types of handicapping conditions and the kinds of adaptations that are necessary, if any.

The following two examples may help participants better to understand exercise programs based on individual goals. If a person wishes to develop muscle strength and endurance in order to compete in wheelchair sports, the choice would be progressive resistance exercises (isotonic exercises or weight-training). If, on the other hand, a disabled person wishes to develop cardiovascular endurance, the choice would be some kind of aerobic exercise.

The following kinds of exercises and training systems are briefly defined. More information on selected exercise programs may be found in Chapter VIII.

Kinds of Exercises: ***

- Aerobics (with oxygen) — any exercise that is vigorous and prolonged, 20-30 minutes or more, which supplies oxygen to the body through cardiorespiratory systems.
- Anaerobics (without oxygen) — any exercise that is not prolonged or sustained in which the oxygen supply to the body is insufficient.
- Calisthenics — any exercise which does not involve the use of barbells and dumbbells or weight-training machines. These exercises may be timed or done to music.
- Isokinetic (dynamic) — any exercise in which the muscle is able to shorten or lengthen to counteract an accommodating resistance developed by a device that allows only a constant rate of movement regardless of the force exerted by a contracting muscle.
- Isometric (static) — any exercise in which the length of the muscle does not shorten during contractions; tension develops, heat is produced, but no mechanical work is performed.
- Isotonic (dynamic) — any exercise in which the muscle is able to contract, shorten or lengthen, and work is performed.
- Progressive Resistance — any exercise used to increase muscle strength by utilizing the overload principle, i.e., subjecting the

---

***Some contemporary physical fitness terminology tends to cause confusion. Although some exercise terms have different names, their functional meaning remains the same.

muscle to a greater-than-normal load.

Training Systems:

- Circuit training — exercises that are individually performed at different stations as the individual moves from one to the other, and there are no rest periods nor periods of decreased activity.
- Interval training — any running or similar physical activity that emphasizes the development of cardiorespiratory endurance. Short distances at near maximal speed are performed and followed by rest intervals or lighter load. This procedure is repeated several times.
- Obstacle course training — physical activities that are individually performed at a number of obstacles formed in a pattern and are challenging in nature. Usually, the individual proceeds from one obstacle to another without stopping.

SIMILARITIES BETWEEN ABLE-BODIED AND HANDICAPPED IN TERMS OF FITNESS NEEDS

The able-bodied and the handicapped have the same fitness needs. It could be said, however, that the handicapped have even a greater need for fitness than do the able-bodied. Not surprisingly, researchers have reported that the disabled are low in all aspects of physical fitness and have the same high risk factors as their able-bodied counterparts: poor nutrition, obesity, high blood pressure, insufficient sleep and rest, use of tobacco, drugs (excluding medication), and alcohol, and lack of physical activity.

Although the literature on physical fitness, physical conditioning, or physical training for the handicapped is rather scarce, what is available reveals quite clearly that their fitness needs are identical to those of the able-bodied population. Like those of their able-bodied counterparts, the disabled fitness needs are cardiovascular endurance, muscle strength, muscular endurance, flexibility or range of motion, weight reduction, if necessary, and, in addition, functional posture correction. The fact that the needs are the same may come as a surprise to many professionals.

Several factors contribute to the low level of physical fitness among handicapped: (1) overeating, (2) sedentary lifestyles, (3) lack of understanding of the concepts of total fitness, (4) lack of early motor development, (5) hereditary qualities, (6) negative attitude toward fitness, (7) negative self-concept and body image, (8) negative attitude toward perspiration, (9) lack of motivation, (10) non-corrective postural problem, (11) fear of failure, (12) lack of access to programs and facilities.

The concept of total fitness is necessary in order that the disabled perform their activities of daily living, become self-dependent, and live healthy and beneficial lives. Each individual has the right to neglect or perpetuate daily healthful living. It is up to the professionals to offer programs and activities in order to promote physical fitness for all handicapped people.

PHYSICAL AND MOTOR FITNESS COMPONENTS: DEFINITIONS

Personnel working with the disabled should familiarize themselves with the five components of physical fitness and the six components of motor fitness. Physical fitness components are closely related to physiological capacity, while motor fitness components have a closer relationship to neurological aspects, i.e., motor ability for performing skills, games or sports.

Physical or Health-Related Fitness Components

- Cardiovascular endurance — the capacity to sustain vigorous physical activity, 20 to 30 minutes or longer, that will increase the supply of oxygen to the heart, lungs and vascular system.
- Muscle strength — the capacity of a muscle to exert a maximal force against resistance.
- Muscle endurance — the capacity of a muscle to exert a force repeatedly over a period of time or to apply strength and sustain it.
- Flexibility — a measure of the range of motion available at a joint or a group of joints performed without undue stress or resistance.

- Body fat composition — the percentage of body weight which is fat.

Motor or Skill-Related Components

- Agility — controlling successive body movements and changing directions quickly and easily.
- Balance — maintaining a specified body position and equilibrium by distributing and controlling the weight of the body.

      Static Balance: holding the body in a
                                stationary position
    Dynamic Balance: holding the body in motion

- Speed — performing rapid successive movements within a short time interval.
- Power — combining strength with speed to perform an explosive type of movement.
- Coordination — performing a complex activity efficiently by stimultaneous use of several muscles or muscle groups.
- Reaction time — perceiving a given stimulus, starting the movement, and completing the movement.

THE RELATIONSHIP OF FITNESS TO SPORTS, RECREATION, ACTIVITIES OF DAILY LIVING, AND THE HEALTH-WELLNESS CONCEPT

Four avenues are identified that may be utilized to develop an adequate level of physical fitness. Each avenue can play an important role in the life of a disabled person, yet each may differ in its approach since individual differences, needs, interests, and aspirations should be considered. Fortunately, the handicapped are beginning to receive a little more attention regarding their educational and personal needs, a fact which hopefully will result in a better and more healthy lifestyle.

Although there is a close relationship between fitness and sports, they differ from each other. "Physical fitness" denotes an improvement in functioning of the heart, lungs, blood vessels and muscles and can be accomplished by aerobic and isotonic exercise. "Sports," on the other hand, denotes the learning of skills and techniques related to a particular sport whereby the individuals seek to gain proficiency in order to improve performance.

Another avenue that a disabled person can use to help maintain an adequate physical fitness level is through participation in recreational types of activities. Recreation is a voluntary activity which can be fun, enjoyable, and pleasurable. It may be organized or unorganized and takes place during the individual's leisure hours. In most cases, the handicapped have an abundance of leisure hours, and offering them organized recreation programs can help to fill their leisure hours in a more productive way. Unorganized recreation, on the other hand, is merely free play whereby the individual chooses the activity he/she wishes to play and usually is not supervised. If the handicapped population were to participate in physical recreation on a regular basis, they would be able to maintain an adequate level of fitness. Social recreation would not offer such benefits, as this kind of recreation is sedentary. The major difference between physical and social recreation is that the former requires physical action, while the latter is passive in nature.

Fitness is essential for carrying out the activities of daily living. The disabled must gain some degree of strength and endurance in order to develop and improve their self-care skills. Obviously, in some cases, this goal can never be accomplished. But without an adequate level of physical fitness, the handicapped person will never achieve independence or even semi-independence. Although some may achieve independence, they will need assistance such as a wheelchair or some other kind of device. Regardless of the type and degree of the disabling condition, physically fit individuals stand a better chance of succeeding in activities of daily living than do unfit persons.

The concept of health-wellness has become very popular with the regular population within recent years but has a long way to go to reach the disabled. Health-wellness, as used here, may be defined as a process whereby people learn and practice good mental and physical health habits. Put in other words, wellness is a combination of good mental and physical fitness, a goal all people should aspire to reach.

Lifestyle, or the way people live, has a profound effect on their mental and physical health. A lifestyle that encompasses sound health practices is inexpensive. In order to live a healthy lifestyle, handicapped individuals must practice good health habits on a daily basis. Most disabled people, like the able-bodied, wish to live a long, healthy and enjoyable life. Actually, this goal is not difficult to reach. The best approach to better health-wellness focuses upon four factors — proper nutrition, ample sleep and rest, efficient stress management, and regular exercise. The disability is not of major concern; the ability one has to pursue the health-wellness avenue to a better life is.

IMPORTANCE OF PHYSICAL FITNESS FOR THE HANDICAPPED

Many handicapped people are capable of walking, jogging, performing calisthenics, and practicing weight-training, all of which can improve their physical fitness level. Depending upon the individual's condition, such activities may need to be adapted. Special Olympics and other special sports programs designed for individuals confined to wheelchairs have stressed physical conditioning and training. The disabled athlete, like any other athlete, must be in top physical shape in order to compete successfully.

The question has been frequently asked, "What difference does it make if the disabled person is not physically fit?" The answer to that question becomes obvious as one analyzes the diseases and problems that confront the handicapped. Among this population, as with the regular population, these diseases and problems are possible: coronary heart disease, hypertension, obesity, diabetes, functional and structural postural difficulties, chronic obstructive lung disease, migraines, insomnia, ulcers, and psychological disorders. To alleviate some of these diseases and problems, it is important to attain and maintain an adequate level of physical fitness. It should be noted, however, that physical fitness is not a panacea, but it does have far-reaching implications physically, emotionally, and psychologically.

Our society breeds an environment of non-fitness. We have fast foods and fast transportation. Admittedly, as a group, for whatever reasons, the disabled have fallen way behind the regular populations with respect to physical fitness because our society has taken away the disabled person's right to self-actualization or because our society has not cared enough to afford them opportunities to learn how to become physically and mentally fit.

In sum, there needs to be a new beginning. Handicapped children, youth, and adults need to be taught sound health and fitness habits. Schools, agencies, institutions, and community recreation departments need to join the fitness movement. The disabled population in particular needs the opportunity to participate in a variety of fitness programs and activities. After all, fitness is for everyone, regardless of age, sex, color, religion, or handicapping condition.

THE CASE FOR TEACHING PHYSICAL FITNESS IN PHYSICAL EDUCATION PROGRAMS

Partly because of P.L. 94-142 and partly because society is beginning to be more concerned about handicapped children and youth, drastic changes are taking place in physical education programs throughout our country. The teaching of mainly motor skills and games is rapidly being replaced by instruction in health-related fitness activities as evidenced by the **Health-Related Physical Fitness Test Manual**, recently published by AAHPERD. Both elementary and secondary school physical-education curriculums are in the process of change. Thus, it seems logical to list the following arguments for the teaching of physical or health-related fitness in physical education programs:

- This is the only way to include health-related fitness into the physical education program.
- Health-related fitness activities can benefit students regardless of their ability level.
- Health-related fitness activities are essential in order for students to undergo the stages of normal physical growth and development.
- Positive attitudes toward health-fitness are formed early in life and should be taught in elementary schools.
- Physical fitness activities and exercise are outlets for couped-up emotions.
- Physical fitness activities can help students to release tensions.
- Students who are physically fit are less injury prone. Physical fitness activities can help to develop strong and healthy bodies.

- Students will have the opportunity to learn the whys, whats, and hows of physical fitness.
- Students can still receive instruction in skills, games, and sports through the health-related instruction approach.

As in any type of instruction in which the focus is on the physical, it is imperative that teachers observe the following precautions:

- Review the medical records.
- Consider the student's disability.
- Avoid giving physical fitness instruction at a fast pace.
- Have daily, weekly, monthly, and yearly instruction plans worked out and organized in advance.
- Be sure the teaching environment is conducive to physical activity and exercise.
- Be sure both the indoor and outdoor facilities are safe.
- Be sure all equipment and supplies are safe to use.
- Know the procedures to follow in case of an accident.

Chapter II

LEARNING ABOUT PHYSICAL ACTIVITY

OVERVIEW OF EXERCISE PHYSIOLOGY

A BRIEF review of exercise physiology seems appropriate at this time as the next chapter will discuss the Stimulus-Organism Response (S.O.R.) Theory which will enable fitness instructors to understand better the functional capabilities of individuals with various handicapping conditions. Exercise physiology is a science that studies what occurs in the human body during exercise. Since exercise involves the entire body, many of the body's systems come under scrutiny.

Basically, there are two types of exercise: aerobics (utilizing oxygen) and anaerobics (not requiring oxygen). All types of physical exercise involve muscle contraction. As muscles contract, they use up energy and produce waste products just as any other system does. Thus, an examination of the various systems of the body — the lungs, heart, and vascular system — must be considered.

Energy sources, such as some food stuffs, and waste products, such as carbon dioxide, are carried from site to site in the body whenever these materials are needed or eliminated. In exercise, a large exchange of materials takes place primarily around the muscles. Exercise physiologists have been studying this phenomenon under a variety of conditions. Consequently, one now knows a considerable amount about what occurs in the body as a result of physical activity.

During strenuous exercise, oxygen transport is increased to offset the oxygen debt created at cellular level. As a response to this increase, the blood vessels get larger and more flexible. The power that drives blood through the transport system is supplied by a muscle pump, the heart. Through intensive study, exercise physiologists have found that the heart responds to physical training just as any other muscle does; it becomes more efficient. The other link in the exercise system consists of the lungs. There gases are exchanged — carbon dioxide is expelled and oxygen is absorbed. Once again, it has been scientifically proven that with training, the lungs get more efficient at processing these gases. All parts of the system improve with use, combining to produce more efficient muscular work at a higher rate and for a longer period of time.

Exercise physiologists have studied all types of physical activity from weight-training to marathon running. Science has reached down to the muscle cell to see what bodily changes actually do take place with exercise. Different changes take place depending on what type of exercise is performed, anaerobic or aerobic. High intensity exercise can take place without the use of oxygen and is called anaerobic work. Glycolysis is an anaerobic process which breaks down glucose, a simple sugar, to two molecules of pyruvic acid. By necessity, the energy used must be derived from a metabolic process that does not require oxygen. This system, however, can be used only for short periods of time. Therefore, the body's capacity for anaerobic work is limited.

Aerobic work requires oxygen and draws on metabolic pathways that can be utilized for extended periods of time. Carbohydrates and fats are used as fuel in this instance. The citric acid cycle utilizes oxygen, an aerobic process, to metabolize pyruvic acid into carbon dioxide.

Much work has been done, however, to try to ascertain if any specific diet would improve training performance. The end result has been that except for highly trained athletes involved in long endurance-type contests, i.e., marathon running, a well-balanced diet yields the best results.

People exercise under all types of environmental conditions, extreme heat, cold, or under water, and at various altitudes. Exercise physiologists have investigated all of these various conditions. As a result, an extensive body of knowledge is now available to people exercising under these varied conditions.

BODY COMPOSITION, WEIGHT CONTROL AND ENERGY BALANCE

There is much emphasis on, and awarenes of, body composition in our modern society, especially now that people are becoming much more fitness conscious. The question that is asked most frequently is, "What is the human body composed of?" The answer is fairly simple. The three major structural body components are muscle, bone, and fat. These components differ when comparing males to females.

Body fat is stored in two different sites within the body as essential fat and storage fat. Essential fat is stored in the marrow of bones and in such organs as the heart, kidneys, liver, lungs, spleen, intestines, brain, spinal cord and lipid-rich tissue throughout the system. This type of fat is required for normal physiological function. Because of certain hormonal functions, females have four times the concentration of this type of fat than do males. Storage fat is in the adipose tissue which accumulates in fat pads and as subcutaneous tissue. It surrounds and protects various organs. Men and women usually have similar distribution of storage fat.

There are numerous methods of assessing body fat composition, but the most effective is underwater weighting. Skin fold calipers and circumference measurements are also commonly used. Body fat varies with sex; females have a 25 percent and males 15 percent.

Obesity may be defined as a state of being overweight by 20 to 250 pounds and is usually caused by overeating. Obese individuals usually have a higher total body fat content, a higher percentage of fat in fat cells, and a higher number of fat cells than do non-obese individuals. Research seems to indicate, however, that obesity is a multi-faceted problem and includes such factors as genetics, environment, and social influences as the major contributors. In addition, modern society is highly mechanized, and people are less active than they used to be; therefore, since fewer calories are burned, they are stored as fat. There are several forms of treatment for obesity, such as diet, medication, and surgery. These treatments have been found to be slightly successful. Even exercise for the obese is difficult and in many cases is bound to fail.

The health risks of obesity are numerous as they correlate

directly with increased incidence of coronary heart disease, hypertension, kidney disease, pulmonary disease, and degenerative joint disease. Therefore, it is extremely important for people to stay within their normal weight limits.

Under normal circumstances, the body does an exquisite job of controlling weight by regulating caloric input and output. To prevent increases in weight and fat, individuals must establish a caloric balance. Basically, there are three energy balance equations:

Caloric intake = energy output ⟶ stable weight
Caloric intake > energy output ⟶ increase weight
Caloric intake < energy output ⟶ decrease weight

Small daily changes in these balances can make dramatic long-term differences. For example, one hundred additional calories over output per day will result in a ten-pound increase of weight per year. A reduction of one hundred calories per day through diet, plus an increase output of one hundred calories per day through exercise can result in a reduction of 21 pounds per year. In short, the combination of a sensible (caloric reduction) diet with regular exercise tends to be the best long-term weight reducing method.

Nutrition is the study of food and how the body utilizes it. Foods are made up of a variety of substances that provide energy. Carbohydrates, fats, and protein are the three main nutrients which provide the necessary energy to maintain body functions both at rest and during exercise.

Carbohydrates are made up of a variety of sugars that serve as the main source for energy and bodily functions. They are broken down into a simple sugar, glucose, which is stored in the muscles and liver and is transported by the blood and utilized by the cells for such activity as muscle contraction. The excess sugar is converted to fat and stored. During exercise, glycogen is used for energy; but as exercise increases, the glycogen storage decreases, and energy is then used from the metabolized fat (converted sugar). If one exercises long enough, the limited glycogen storage is used.

The second nutrient, fat, has many forms, such as simple, compound, saturated, unsaturated, and derived. Fats provide the body with a large storage of energy during rest and exercise. Fat in the body also provides protection to vital organs.

Protein is the third nutrient that provides the body with necessary energy to maintain proper functioning. Proteins are the basic structural substance of each cell and are made up of amino acids. The body needs 20 amino acids to function properly. Sources of protein are meats, fish, eggs, and milk. Like carbohydrates, the excess of calories in protein is converted to fat.

Nutrition is an important factor in relation to exercise or physical activity. Energy is supplied by nutrients in the foods we eat, i.e., fats, carbohydrates, proteins, aided by minerals and vitamins. Fats contain 9 calories per gram; carbohydrates, 4 calories per gram; and protein, 4 calories per gram. Carbohydrates, which are contained in 50 percent of everyone's diet, are broken into simple sugar or glucose, which the body uses as its primary source of energy. Proteins are organic compounds that are needed to build and repair body tissues. Minerals are important components of the body; calcium, for example, aids in the formation of bones and teeth. Vitamins are not a source of energy, but they help to absorb and metabolize other nutrients needed by the body.

Energy is derived from such sources as food, mechanical function, and chemical reactions of the body that provide strength and endurance and enable the human body to move. There are many factors that influence energy needs, such as body size, age, type and amount of daily activity. The measurement of energy is expressed in calories, or the amount of heat required to raise the temperature of 1 kg. (2.2 lb.) of water to 1°. A certain amount of energy must be utilized to maintain certain vital functions — respiration, heart contraction, and other metabolic activities. The utilization of energy at rest is called the basal metabolic rate (BMR), a rate which varies in each individual. The **basal metabolic rate** can be determined by measuring oxygen consumption during resting periods. Since oxygen is used by the body to release energy from food products, oxygen uptake is equal to the amount of energy the body utilizes.

As people grow older, the basal metabolic rate goes down five to ten percent every ten years. This decrease, in addition to lack of exercise, decrease in activity, and a sedentary lifestyle, may lead to obesity.

Food ingested and activity performed have an effect on energy expenditure. Calories in food are transformed into energy through digestion, absorption, and biochemical reaction of various nutrients.

The amount of calories varies in different foods, thus energy levels also vary. The caloric value can be determined if we know the composition and weight of the food.

Climate also affects the basal metabolic rate. The body works harder in heat to maintain body equilibrium. In cold weather, a lean person burns more calories than an obese person does. The extra weight carried by an obese person works as an insulator against cold, whereas a thin person will shiver.

As previously mentioned, oxygen is used by the body to release energy from food products. Through sustained activity, energy is released through the transportation of oxygen to the cells. The breathing process, or pulmonary ventilation, is the method by which oxygen is absorbed. Oxygen is dissolved in the blood and combines with hemoglobin, the iron portion molecule of the red blood cell. When oxygen combines with hemoglobin, it increases the blood-carrying capacity 65-70 times that which is dissolved in the fluid portion. During heavy exercise, the hemoglobin gives up 75 percent of its oxygen to supply working cells. Physical activity affects oxygen consumption and carbon dioxide production more than any other metabolic stress. During light and moderate exercise, ventilation increases with oxygen uptake; and during more intense exercise, ventilation takes a sharp upswing.

POSTURE AND BODY MECHANICS

Posture and proper body alignment are important for movement and body mechanics. Posture deviations are classified as "structural," referring to permanent change, and "functional," referring to temporary changes involving muscles and ligaments. Individuals maintain certain body positions that become habitual while walking, sitting, standing, and exercising. What they may find as a comfortable position may not be the proper body alignment. The neuromuscular system responds to these incorrect positions.

Awareness of kinesthetic sense and balance are also factors that help to develop posture and the proper body positions. Some handicapping conditions may make it difficult for an individual to maintain the proper body positions and posture because of contracting muscles, improper balance, lack of awareness of kinesthetic sense, and a limited range of motion.

Poor functional posture cannot be corrected by performing a few minutes of exercise three times a week. The neuromuscular system must be retrained over a period of time in order to establish good body alignment and mechanics. Good posture development should be continuous each day and should be controlled to produce the best results in strength, flexibility, efficiency of movement, and relaxation. Some handicapping conditions make it difficult for the individual to move efficiently and to control his/her neuromuscular system.

STRESS AND ITS EFFECT
ON THE HANDICAPPED

Stress is a term with multiple meanings. For some people it refers to unpleasant things that happen to them, while others use the word to describe the physical or mental tension they feel when unpleasant events occur. Neither of these meanings is sufficient in and of itself. Stress needs to be considered as a complex process by which events occur; they are appraised and interpreted by the individual, and the person responds at both a psychological and physiological level.

The events, commonly referred to as "stressors," can be environmental or psychological. To the extent that handicapped individuals live in a society that negatively values deviancy, they may be expected to incur an excessive number of such stressors. Lack of accessibility to public buildings, negative societal attitudes, transportation difficulties, and lack of employment opportunities are examples of the unique environmental stressors that handicapped individuals are subjected to.

The handicapped individual's appraisal of stress concerns itself with an assessment of how dangerous the events are and whether the resources are present that will allow the individual to cope in an adaptive fashion. Because of the self-esteem difficulties that are frequently present in handicapped individuals, these persons may be more likely to perceive events as dangerous and in turn be more likely to conclude than do the non-handicapped that they do not have the ability to cope adequately. Lack of perceived control and lack of social support because of stigmatization associated with the handicap may lead handicapped individuals to make appraisals that are much more catastrophic than warranted. Because handicapped individuals may, in fact, lack the resources necessary to cope with stress, such as lack of mobility and reduced financial resources because of high medical costs, they may conclude that they are not able to cope. Feelings of helplessness are a natural consequence of such conclusions. If either catastrophic appraisals or feelings of helplessness persist, handicapped individuals will be at risk for the development of stress-related disorders such as headaches, low back pain, and hypertension. Such feelings are also likely to result in poor lifestyle habits including poor nutrition, inadequate exercise, tobacco usage, and excessive alcohol use.

At the response level, the actual handicap itself may influence the person's reaction at either a psychological or physiological level. At a psychological level, stress is manifested as worry, mental anxiety, irritability, sleep difficulties, low frustration tolerance and depression. Physiological reactions include dilated pupils, tight throat, tense neck and upper back, shallow breathing, fast pulse rate, and cool, perspiring hands. To the extent that the handicapped individual may encounter excessive stressors and be unable to cope with them adequately, the issue of stress management becomes crucial.

Successful stress management involves intervening at each of three levels, i.e., helping handicapped individuals change environmental conditions that are serving as a source of stress, providing individuals with cognitive coping strategies that will allow them to make more realistic appraisals and, lastly, exposing them to the myriad of self-regulation techniques that are currently available to deal with the physiological effects of stress. Such techniques include biofeedback, exercise, meditation, yoga, relaxation training, stress innoculation training, and autogenic therapy.

The use of these techniques with handicapped individuals requires a sound knowledge of the nature of restrictions associated with the handicap. Self-regulation strategies should be selected based on their appropriateness for the individual client. While meditative exercises might be most appropriate for individuals who are able to maintain effortless concentration over an extended period of time, physical (active) exercise would perhaps be appropriate for individuals who have trouble concentrating and who need to be on the go in order to be happy. In any case, stress management is a trial and error process, and techniques should not be arbitrarily assigned to individuals without knowledge as to the personality dynamics of the individual and the physical parameters of the handicap.

Chapter III

UNDERSTANDING THE FUNCTIONAL CAPABILITIES OF THE HANDICAPPED

A T the outset, two basic questions need to be answered: First, who are the handicapped? And second, what approach has proven successful in teaching physical fitness activities to this special population?

As part of the answer to the first question, personnel working with the handicapped should become acquainted with three terms which society usually associates with this segment of the population. Although the three terms are used interchangeably and synonymously, they do elicit specific connotations when analyzed closely. The contemporary trend, however, is to view the special population as people rather than label, classify, or place them into specific categories.

In this text, as mentioned previously, the terms handicapped and disabled are used interchangeably. However, it seems advisable, at this juncture, to point out the differences among the three terms frequently used by physicians, educators, and lay persons. Furthermore, the three terms, as defined below, are used as "descriptors."*

Impairments refer to conditions which, either observable or diagnosed, affect a specific area of the body or body part(s). These conditions may be organic or functional. They may or may not keep persons from functioning adequately or up to capacity. Impairments can be either permanent or temporary. Permanent impairing conditions include amputations, brain damage, cerebral palsy, or birth

---

*Adapted from Julian U. Stein, "Perceptual-Motor Development of Handicapped Children- Thoughts, Observations, and Questions," *Foundations and Practices in Perceptual-Motor Learning — A Quest for Understanding.* Washington, American Association for Health Physical Education, and Recreation, 1971, p. 29.

defects. Temporary impairing conditions include functional speech defects, emotional problems, social maladjustments, and specific motor deficiencies.

Disabilities refer to conditions that, because of impairments, may keep persons from performing up to their capabilities. These people may also be limited in physical, mental, psychological, or intellectual capacities, or any combination of these. Individuals with disabling conditions may not be able to perform specific tasks, skills, or activities safely or adequately. All so-called disabled individuals should be encouraged to participate in some type of fitness activity or program. For example, a below-the-elbow amputee can develop overall muscular strength and endurance by weight training.

Handicaps refers to conditions that, because of impairment or disability, affect persons psychologically, emotionally, socially, or any combination of these. Since many individuals with impairing or disabling conditions do not consider themselves to be handicapped by their conditions, they adjust very well. It is the attitude of society that often labels them as such.

Fitness instructors need to have a working knowledge of the various types of handicapping or impairing conditions. As it is not the intent of this chapter to provide such a comprehensive treatment, readers should refer to the book noted below.*

The answer to the second question, concerning what approach has proven successful in teaching physical fitness activities to special populations, is the main reason this chapter was written. It is intended to provide the fitness instructor with a teaching approach that has proven effective. Once instructors familiarize themselves with the various types of handicapping conditions, the foundation will have been laid for understanding the functional capacities of handicapped persons.

Authorities in the field of special education have recognized the need for the development of Individualized Educational Programs (IEP's). Through design and implementation IEP's require:

- Identification of the individual's strengths and weaknesses
- Establishment of individual goals and objectives
- Development and evaluation of an appropriate IEP.

---

*Arthur G. Miller and James V. Sullivan, *Teaching Physical Activities to Impaired Youth: An Approach to Mainstreaming*, (New York: John Wiley and Sons, 1982).

If physical fitness activities are to be meaningful and valuable to the participant, the instructor must utilize a process similar to the IEP to develop an Individualized Fitness Activity Program (IFAP). However, before instructors can individualize their fitness programs, they must be aware of following important considerations for teaching the disabled:*

- Persons who have specific sensory deficiencies, such as blindness, partial sight, deafness, and partial hearing, are affected primarily at the input or sensory level; they will have difficulty in receiving and transmitting stimuli.
- Mentally retarded people are affected primarily at levels in which information and data are collected, indexed, stored, and made available for use through interpretation and integration. Their major difficulty is associating mental aspects to the total sensory-motor process.
- Persons with neurological problems such as brain damage and cerebral dysfunctions are usually affected at different levels in the sensory motor process, depending upon what section of the brain and nervous system is involved. For example, an emotionally disturbed individual may be affected at any level.
- Physically handicapped persons are affected primarily at the output or performance level, where information and data are translated into motor activity. These persons will have difficulty in performing specific movements.
- Some handicapped people may have problems at several levels; these multiple conditions are more severe and difficult to remediate in terms of providing such participants with fitness activities and programs.

In addition to the five important considerations discussed above, fitness instructors should acquaint themselves with four major senses involved in the performance of motor acts. These same four senses have been described as follows:**

Tactual or Tactile Sense. The tactual sense, the sense of touch, enables people to differentiate between objects on the basis of size, texture, or design. Sensory end organs in the skin located all over the body enable individuals to feel variations in direct pressure to the body surface. Those areas involved in fine motor tasks, such as the

*Julian U. Stein, *op. cit.*, p. 30.
**Unpublished material, author unknown, n.d.

THE HUMAN BRAIN

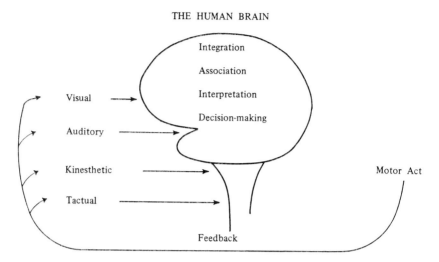

hands, have a high concentration of tactual receptors. These receptors, once stimulated, send their message back to the spinal cord, then upward to the brain.

Kinesthetic Sense. Kinesthesis is the sensory modality which allows people to "feel" a movement. It provides them with an awareness of body parts, their positions, and the direction of their movements. It is the sense relied upon for information when individuals move with their eyes closed. For example, bringing the tips of the index fingers together over the head with the eyes closed is accomplished only with the aid of kinesthesis. The sensory receptors for kinesthesis are located in muscles, muscle tendons, and around the joints. They are stimulated by stretch, tension, or pressure and send their messages back to the brain via the spinal cord.

Auditory Sense. Hearing is initiated by sound waves disrupting air outside the ear. As these vibrations come in contact with the ear drum, they set it in motion. The drum, as it vibrates, acts upon three bones in the middle ear — stirrup, anvil, and hammer — and they, in turn, vibrate. This vibration is then transmitted to the inner ear where a fluid contained in the cochlea (a snail-like structure) picks up the vibration. At this point, the waves moving through this fluid in the channels of the cochlea set little hair-like structures (cilia) moving in undulating fashion. These undulations result in a nervous impulse which is then relayed via the auditory nerve to the hearing centers in the brain. This admittedly over-simplified description of the hearing apparatus illustrates the complexity associated with the auditory sense.

Visual Sense. The visual mechanism is initiated by light rays passing through the pupil of the eye and focusing on the retina. This process sets up nerve impulses which are conducted via the optic nerve back to the visual cortex. The light energy to nervous impulses is beyond the scope of this discussion.

One of the interesting factors associated with the visual sense is that it is the most unreliable of the senses. Optical illusions such as the one in which people "see" water collected on the surface of the road as they drive on a sunny day exemplify the ease with which people can be fooled through the visual modality.

The best approach to use to determine the functional capabilities of the handicapped is the Stimulus-Organism-Response Theory. From the instructors' point of view, this theory will take into account the personal interests and expectations of the handicapped participant. Yet, desirable as individualized instruction is, one other criterion is urged. Both the sensory and the motor capacity of the participant should be weighed against the sensory and motor requirements of the proposed fitness activity.

In the simplified schema for developing an effective IFAP presented below, the relationship between an assigned activity, a handicapped person, and that individual's performance is represented in classical psychological terms of the S-O-R theory.

S (Stimulus)	O (Organism)	R (Response)
Identifiable external factor	Unobservable sensory and motor capacity of the handicapped individual	Observable response associated with the activity

Though generalized, this schema has many applications, especially for instructors of the handicapped. On the following pages is a detailed explanation of the S-O-R series as a means of selecting an appropriate physical fitness activity. These guidelines should be useful to instructors in assessing the person's degree and quality of response.

Stimulus (S): Within the above schema, a **stimulus** refers to any agent or environment change factor which the person experiences sensorially that directly influences activity. As used here, the stimulus is produced by the activity and the capacity of the individual to appropriately experience it. Such a stimulus may be quantitative or qualitative or both. For example, **verbal** instructions (auditory), **visual** instructions, **tactile** instructions by touch and **kinesthetic**, feedback through muscles, tendons, and joints and **vestibular**, feedback through body orientation or balance are all sensory or information input sources. What needs to be determined is the sensory requirements of learning and the capacity to perform a physical fitness activity.

Organism (O): Organism refers to all aspects of the individual that intervene between the Stimulus and Response. This would include not only the individual's ability to interpret the (S) but also his/her ability to determine the appropriate (R) to the (S). In most cases the sensory and motor capacities of an individual (O) are inferred by relating in identifiable stimulus (S) to an associated and observable response (R). A notable exception would involve the lack of a sensory or motor organ. Usually, however, a handicapped person has a diminished capacity rather than a total absence of it. For example, because of a person's brain damage, his/her (S) may be inappropriately interpreted and thus lead to an inappropriate response.

Response (R): All voluntary responses (R) occur in association with stimuli (S). The goal of the instructor is to elicit the appropriate voluntary response through the utilization of an identifiable stimulus. An inappropriate or diminished response may indicate any one or more of the following conditions: the stimulus (S) is inappropriate for eliciting the desired response (R); a sensory deficiency or motor deficiency (O), or both, exists; the organism (O) is incapable of accomplishing the response (R). For the purposes of this schema, the response is restricted to voluntary motor behavior that is observable.

All physical fitness activities involve a complex series of S-O-R. For example, although verbal instructions (auditory stimuli) may be utilized in teaching weight training, the participant is also learning from visual, tactile, and kinesthetic senses. Thus, this particular activity may involve all of the sensory system.

The response requirements are often as complex as the stimulus. For example, in walking, a person is required not only to move the legs but also to position the feet and the toes, and to change balance and body position.

The first step in determining the appropriateness of a physical fitness activity is to identify the stimuli and responses required of both the participant and the activity. The second step involves identifying the limits of the individual (O) that would negate the appropriate association of a stimulus with a response. For example, although a learning impaired individual may not possess S and R limits, there are definite O limitations. In order to associate S and R, the instructor may have to reduce these to their component parts i.e. the verbal instructions (S) need to be simplified or less complex and require only partial responses (R).

Generally speaking, the more substantially handicapped the person, the more detailed the IFAP should be. Although the instructor may not view the detailed IFAP as necessary, it is imperative that it be completely developed to assure that the activity is appropriate to the individual's functioning capabilities. Further, the IFAP assures that the instructor has explored various avenues open to the participant. For example, until it was realized that verbal (auditory) instruction could replace visual feedback, skiing was considered an inappropriate activity for the blind.

Another physical activity performed by the blind is fencing. When performing this activity, participants utilize a variety of stimuli including body orientation (vestibular), muscles, joints and tendons (kinesthetic), and hearing (auditory). The key point that instructors need to become aware of is that all physical or motor activities consist of a variety of stimuli. The instructor needs to identify the stimuli so as to enable the participant to learn how to perform the activity.

In order that fitness instructors better understand the S-O-R theory, a hypothetical case is presented utilizing its schema. The illustration is divided into three parts: background information, analysis of the S-O-R training process: teaching a mentally retarded child how to walk, and interpretation. It should be noted that although the primary mode of instruction in this situation is verbal (auditory), visual, tactile, kinesthetic and vestibular sensory systems also play a role. Moreover, other physical fitness activities such as jogging, weight training, swimming, aerobic dancing, cycling, and calisthenics can utilize the S-O-R teaching process. Instructors, however, need to take the necessary time to analyze each stimulus and response associated with a particular activity and develop a teaching strategy which will permit the handicapped person a better opportunity to learn and to succeed.

Background Information

Capacity of the Individual: John, an eight-year-old moderately mentally retarded child, is capable of standing in a "walker," but shows no capacity for moving his feet forward or backward. He can creep by coordinating hand and leg movements and he can sit without support. He has no visual or auditory problems. Such evidence suggests that in spite of his development lag, John could be taught how to walk.

Stimulus Capacity: John follows simple, short-sentence, oral directions; therefore, auditory stimuli associated with walking will be offered as the primary mode of instruction. However, the instructor must bear in mind that there is also visual, tactile, kinesthetic, and vestibular interaction.

Response Capacity: John's present motor ability indicates that he has made some progress on the developmental scale from creeping to standing unaided in a walker. Moreover, while standing in a walker, he is capable of lifting one foot at a time.

S-R Relationship: While standing in a walker, John is capable of responding to simple directions, "Lift your left foot."

Activity Goal: The short-term goal is to develop basic walking itself; this will involve John's stepping forward while standing in the walker. The long-term goal is to increase his ambulation through walking so as to develop his cardiovascular endurance and, in time, enable him to run and play games.

From the above background information, John's capacities have been established and a goal has been set. Considering John's present capacities, the stimulus (S) and response (R) have been identified and placed in a developmental sequence. In the chart that follows, the analysis of the activity (walking) starts at John's present functioning level.

Interpretation

Stimuli: Ten different stimuli (verbal instructions) and their relationship to a desired response have been identified in the preced-

An Analysis of the S-O-R Training Process
Teaching a Mentally Retarded Child to Walk

STIMULUS	EXPLANATION	S-R RELATIONS
1. Lift your **left** foot, put it down (S_1).	John has shown the ability to respond to these **separate** directions when they are given **simultaneously** with the activity.	Two separate stimuli ("lift and put down") associated with two separate responses (lift and put down the foot).
2. Lift your **right** foot, put it down (S_2).		
3. Lift your **left** foot, put it down (S_3).	Instruction given **prior** to total activity.	One stimulus (instruction) associated with one response (activity).
4. Lift your **right** foot, put it down (S_4).	Instruction given **prior** to total activity.	
5. Lift your **left** foot, put it down/lift your **right** foot, put it down (S_5).	S_3 and S_4 are associated (a) S_5-instructions (S_3 then S_4) given **prior** to the appropriate sequence (lift the right foot).	Two separate stimuli (S_3 and S_4) associated with two separate responses (activities). One stimulus (instruction) associated with one response (activity).
6. Lift your **left** foot, put it down/lift your **right** foot, put it down (S_6).	(b) S_6-instruction (S_3 and S_4) given **prior** to total activity.	

STIMULUS	EXPLANATION	S-R RELATIONS
7. Lift your **left** foot, put it forward, put it down (S_7).	A new stimulus ("put it forward") is placed between two known effective stimuli. Instructions are given **simultaneously** with each movement of the total activity. This activity presents a special problem in that S_8 must follow S_7 unless an intermediary step (returning left foot) is introduced.	Six separate stimuli (S_7 and S_8) associated with six separate responses.
8. Lift your **right** foot, put it forward, put it down (S_8).		
9. Lift your **left** foot, put it forward, put it down/lift your **right** foot, put it forward, put it down (S_9).	**S_7 and S_8 are associated** Instruction S_7 and S_8 given **prior** to appropriate sequence (left foot then right foot).	Two stimuli (S_7 and S_8) associated with two responses.
10. Lift your **left** foot, put it forward, put it down, lift your **right** foot, put it forward, put it down (S_{10}).	Instruction given **prior** to total activity.	One stimulus (instruction) associated with one activity.

ing chart. The initial stimuli have been selected for their appropriateness to John's diminished response-level.

Complexity is increased by changing the relationship of an effective stimulus to an associated response, or by combining stimuli, or even by adding a new stimulus to known effective stimuli. For example, S_3 and S_4 (see chart) represent a change in the S-R relationship resulting from the previous stimuli (S_1 and S_2); S_5 represents the combining of S_3 and S_4; S_7 and S_8 represent the addition of new stimuli to already effective stimuli.

Responses: The required responses are identified by the S (verbal instructions).

The effectiveness of the analysis of S-R, above, can only be established by applying it to a specific "organism" (John). This process determines whether the identified S's and R's are appropriate; if inappropriate, changes will be required. Example:

> **S_1 and S_2**: John can raise his feet in response to simple instructions. If the appropriate responses are made, S_3 follows.
>
> **S_3**: John can complete the required activity (lift and put down appropriate foot). If the appropriate response (R) is not obtained, S_3 should be reexamined. A deficiency in S_3 may reflect a deficiency in the S-R relationship. If the relationship is not learned after a reasonable number of repeated instructions, an intermediary stimulus between S_1 and S_3 must be looked for, or a new stimulus introduced.
>
> **S_5**: This represents a combining of S_3 and S_4, which John has already responded to separately.
>
> **S_7 and S_8**: The stimuli complex adds a number of potential problems. A new stimulus "put your foot forward" is inserted in an effort to produce the desired response. Furthermore, it has not been determined whether or not the new stimulus, "put your foot foward," will elicit this required response. By presenting the stimulus **simultaneously** with the required response, a number of S's and R's are, in essence, combined. At this step in the process, John can appropiately respond to all S's with the exception of "put your foot forward."

Although this S-O-R series may appear complex, it is relatively simple if the goal of the activity is an observable motor response. Furthermore, through trial and error, the instructor can quickly establish the capacity level of the child. For example, the first time through the sequence John may have been capable of responding from S_1 through S_8.

Instructing the handicapped to participate in a physical fitness activity requires an understanding of both the individual and the activity. It should be noted here that the S-O-R theory can be utilized regardless of a person's sensory and/or motor deficiencies. This approach is effective with the verbal, the visual, the tactile, and the kinesthetic sensory input approaches to instruction. But to apply the S-O-R process successfully, the instructor must analyze the problems and develop a clear and orderly sequence of instructions. In addition, he/she must teach with patience, cheer, and adaptability to challenges.

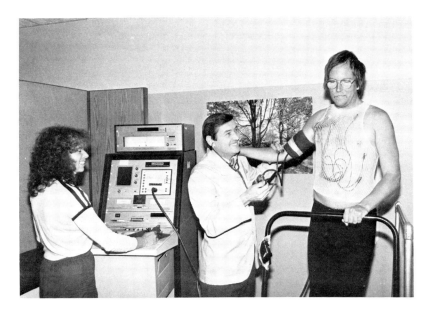

Figure 1. The graded exercise test.

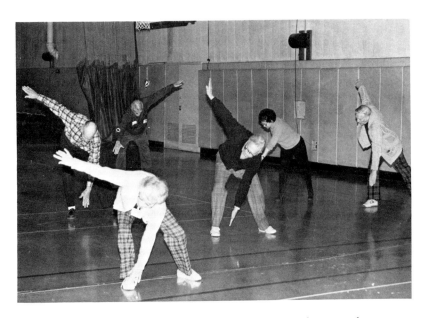

Figure 2. A flexibility exercise is performed by a pulmonary class.

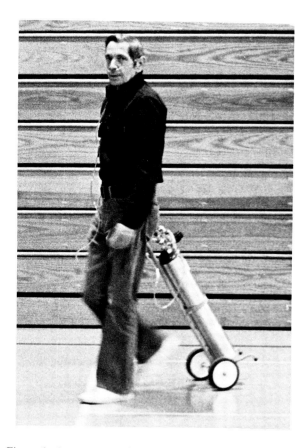

Figure 3. An oxygen tank does not interfere with walking.

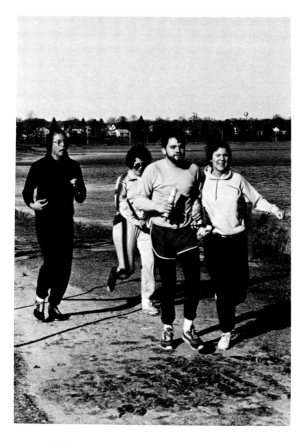

Figure 4. Jogging can be enjoyed by all.

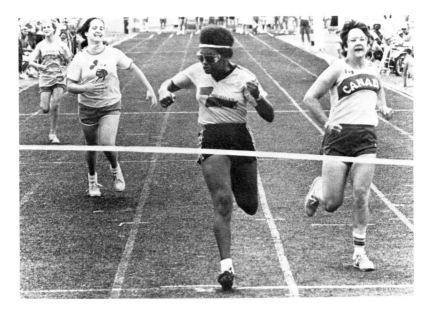

Figure 5. Becoming fit means enjoying competition.

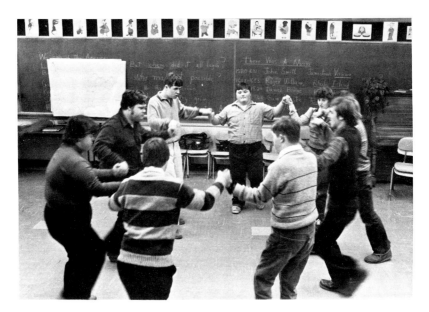

Figure 6. Dancing is a good activity for developing cardiovascular endurance.

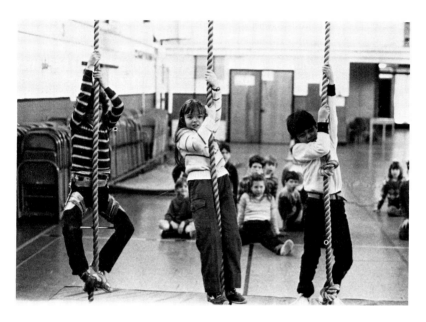

Figure 7. Rope climbing helps develop upper body strength.

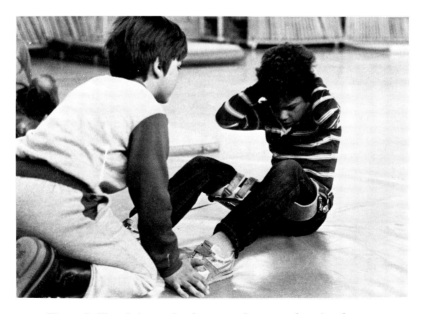

Figure 8. Timed sit-ups develop muscular strength and endurance.

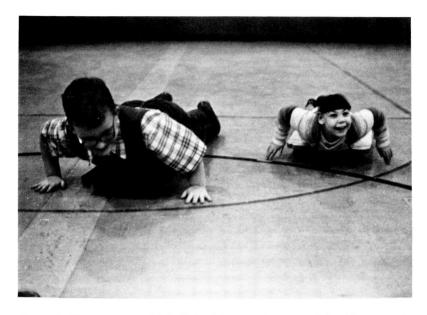

Figure 9. Gym scooter activities help children gain arm and shoulder strength.

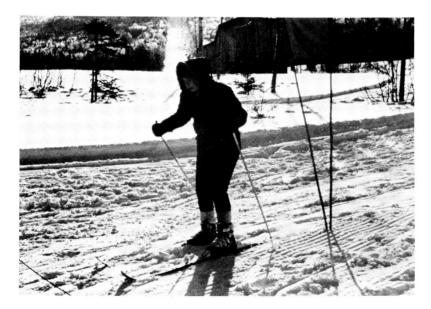

Figure 10. Cross country skiing can help increase cardiovascular endurance.

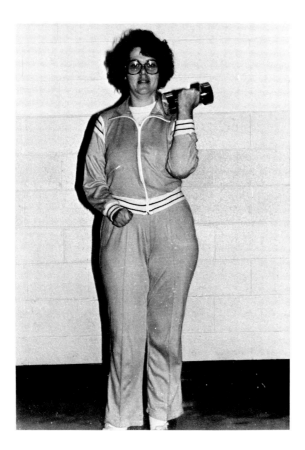

Figure 11. A participant with cerebral palsy performs bicep curls.

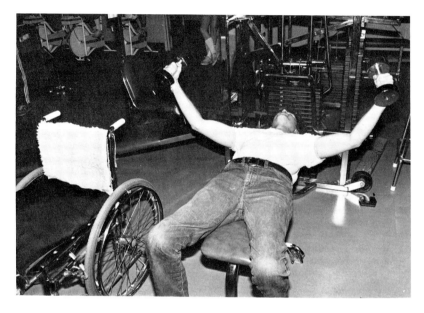

Figure 12. The "flyer" is a good activity for developing the chest muscles.

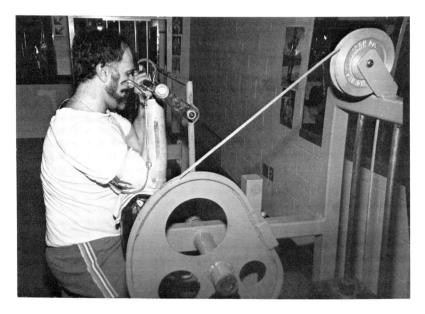

Figure 13. A forearm amputee performs bicep curls on a weight training machine.

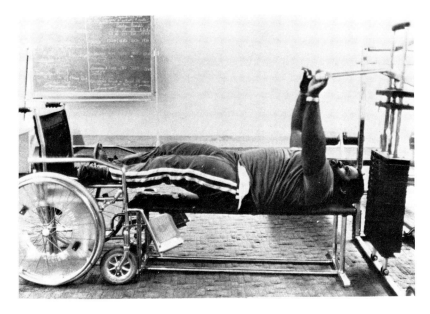

Figure 14. A bench press is performed on a Universal weight training machine

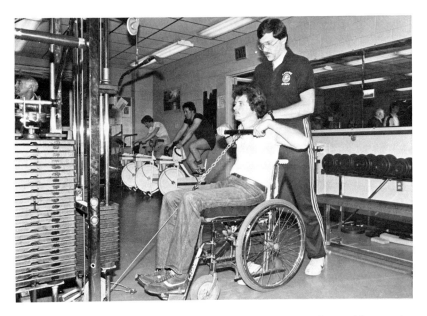

Figure 15. A paraplegic receives assistance in order to perform a bicep curl.

Part II

ORGANIZATION AND ADMINISTRATION
OF FITNESS PROGRAMS
FOR THE HANDICAPPED

Chapter IV

ESTABLISHING FITNESS GOALS AND OBJECTIVES

A N integral part of an effective planning process is establishing goals and objectives. Planning should involve all fitness personnel so that both short-term and long-term plans may be formulated. When goals and objectives are clearly defined, a more definitive description of needs and services is possible. Thus, in the discussion that follows, three types of goals and objectives related to physical fitness for the handicapped will be identified.

There are differences between goals and objectives. Goals are general statements of purpose. They are expressed in terms of desired results or outcomes, indicating why activities are performed. Usually goals are achieved over a long period of time, extending anywhere from one year to five years. As part of the planning process, they should be reviewed annually, but not necessarily changed. A goal is analogous to a high-rise building, in that there are many steps before a desired floor is reached. Just as each floor reached indicates progress, so objectives serve as indices as to how much has been accomplished.

Objectives are statements that are measurable, observable behavior that leads toward a goal. Whereas goals have an indeterminate life span, objectives define time limits precisely. Objectives lend concrete reality to what are often vague hopes that are contained in goal statements. They allow handicapped people to define experiences that can measurably determine whether there is movement toward a goal. A well-stated objective will provide specific guidelines for participant, instructor, and program and will clarify what each of these must do to reach desired goals. There are both goals and objectives for the participant, the instructor, and the program. The selection of objectives should always be in accordance with the instructor's and the participant's capabilities as well as with the resources available for conducting the program.

SETTING GOALS: AN OPPORTUNITY FOR CREATIVE THINKING

The day-to-day tasks involved in organizing and administering fitness programs for handicapped people and students leave little time for thinking ahead to determine what needs to be accomplished. Goals that seem to be unrealistic at present may become real possibilities in the future. Goal setting can release the creative energies of both instructors and administrators; therefore, effective planning can translate into reality.

Fitness instructors support goals that reflect their creative thinking. If goal setting does not bring about the hopes and desires of the group, the end product will be only definitions of what is already being done. Goals will move fitness instructors, participants, and programs to a higher level of functioning.

One approach to stimulate visionary thinking might be as follows:

- Prepare the instructional staff for a few sessions in creative thinking and have their permission to engage in brainstorming as a group.
- Tell the members to relax so that they do not feel pressured.
- Ask the question, "What could be happening at school or at a particular establishment one year from now if really positive changes occur?"
- Ask the members to visualize concrete events that could happen. They should be specific about what they foresee happening among the instructors, participants, and programs.
- Have the group list the images that they perceive individually; then share them with the entire group.
- Write all the ideas on a large white easel pad so that all may see.

- Identify the concepts that seem to be similar or in the same general area. Have the members select at least four or five concepts that could be translated into goals.

Steps for Defining Goals

Although many goals are implicit as they relate to instructors, participants, and programs, the selection of a few explicit, commonly-held goals helps to focus energies, exercise creative behavior, and develop imagination. Goals provide a challenge to see beyond current demands and identify the values inherent in them. Once the instructors and administrators agree to meet a few times, they can clarify goals and create a future-oriented climate within the group.

There are six specific steps that might be utilized when defining goals:

- Several meetings must be held which all fitness instructors are required to attend. In school settings, all interested personnel should attend.
- At these meetings, each member must come up with a list of items that are to be written on a large white easel pad. An "S" is placed beside items that are similar or quite similar; an "R" is placed beside items that refer to the same issue; a "G" is placed beside items that fall into the same general area.
- For the purpose of clarity, each person attending the meetings may ask questions of other members. The group leader then goes through the complete list with all members to note which of the items are similar to others, and to what degree.
- The group then identifies those items that are most common. These are listed on another page in summary form that is agreed to by the group.
- After listing the four or five issues that are most common, they are rank-ordered by the group, through discussion, in terms of the greatest importance.
- The issues are refined and restated as goals.

Goals of the Participant

To increase range of motion
To gain more over-all flexibility

To improve functional muscular strength
To improve muscular endurance
To improve cardiovascular endurance
To establish an acceptable social and emotional relationship
To participate in Special Olympics or Wheelchair sports

Goals of the Instructor

To obtain knowledge in exercise physiology and kinesiology related to the handicapped
To learn about handicapping conditions
To become informed about methods and techniques of fitness testing related to the handicapped
To study the methods and techniques for leading or teaching fitness activities to handicapped individuals
To acquire information on how to use adaptations with physical fitness activities
To gather information so as to provide fitness counseling to handicapped individuals

Goals of the Program

To offer appropriate adapted physical fitness activities so as to increase participation
To provide competent leaders or teachers
To develop standards for each fitness activity offered
To offer an effective adapted fitness program based on facilities and equipment
To establish rules governing vertical and horizontal organizational communications
To set up procedures for evaluation

DEVELOPING GOOD OBJECTIVES

When determining objectives, one should ask the following questions:

• What observations will show that progress is being made toward a goal?

- What observations will show that there is digression from a goal?
- What can be done to reach a goal within the capabilities of the instructor and participants and with the resources available for the program?

Poor objectives can lead to confusion and undermine a group's intention to accomplish a goal. A poor objective tends to increase ambiguity rather than reduce it.

A good objective considers four questions:

- What will be accomplished?
- Who and what will be measured?
- When will the measurement take place?
- How much progress toward the standard has been reached?

"What" refers to the action to be completed; "who" and "what" refer to the instructor, the participant, and the program; "when" refers to a specific date; and "how much" refers to some standard or quality to be achieved.

Steps for Defining Objectives

- After faculty/staff have agreed on four or five goal statements, they should now focus on one goal at at time.
- The group must ask the question, "What objectives must be accomplished if this goal is to be reached?" There will be many answers, and they should be written on a large, white easel pad.
- After completing the previous step, the group looks at the variety of answers and selects several of them using the following criteria:

> Is this an important change?
> Is it measurable?
> Can it be observed in some way?
> Is it an indicator of the goal?

- The small list that results from the previous step will become the **what** of one or more objectives. At this time the group should begin to identify the **who** and **what** for which the objective is defined.
- Now the **when** should be considered. It may be reasonable to

define a target date at this time. It is often more useful, however, to delay setting a target date until objectives are clarified in order to allow enough time for everything to get done.

- Defining the **how much** part of the progress toward an objective may involve expert advice on evaluation. It also means that the faculty/staff must reach a consensus on reasonable expectations from the instructor, the participant, and the program. The following procedures may prove helpful:
- Brainstorm ideas about evaluations and expectations. These ideas should be written down.
- Select some persons who are familiar with evaluation and measurement to work with the group.
- Define and rework the ideas, clarify measurement procedures and expectations, and have the group discuss the well-formed objectives at another meeting.
- When objectives are completed and agreed upon, review all of the objectives for clarity and reasonableness, making any adjustments that are necessary.

Objectives of the Participant

To increase movements by rotating, bending and extending all functional body parts (specified number)

To increase bending, stretching and twisting exercises (specified number)

If possible, to perform the basic weight-training exercises and/or alternates three times a week according to functional ability

To perform some type of aerobic activity at least three times a week, for at least thirty minutes or longer

To train at least three times a week for a particular sport

To attain an acceptable physical fitness level through exercise, games, or sports

According to intelligence, to understand the effects of exercise on the body

When possible, to alleviate or reduce the handicapping condition

According to intelligence, to understand better the handicapping condition

To learn how to release tension and stress
To learn how to relax by exercising
To strive for social and emotional acceptance
According to intelligence, to learn what constitutes a healthy lifestyle

Objectives of the Instructor

To attend workshops, symposia, or conferences on fitness leadership
To read books and periodicals on the subjects
To register for unversity or college courses in physiology of exercise and kinesiology
To attend workshops, symposia, or conferences on handicapping conditions
To read books and periodicals on the subject
To visit fitness programs where testing is done
To attend workshops, symposia, or conferences on fitness testing
To read books and periodicals on the subject
If available, to take a university or college course on fitness evaluation
If available, to read books and periodicals that deal with methods and techniques for leading or teaching fitness activities to the handicapped
If available, to review literature dealing with various ways to adapt and/or accommodate handicapped individuals in various kinds of physical fitness activities
To visit fitness programs for the handicapped where counseling is provided for the participants

Objectives of the Program

To design the program in such a way as to encourage participation
To provide specific criteria for each adapted physical fitness activity offered
To provide training in leading or teaching fitness activities
To provide realistic standards for each fitness activity offered

To provide facilities and equipment, either on site or in the community, which meet the needs of the program

To provide a program which offers the staff or faculty opportunities for interpersonal communications as well as communication with administrators

To conduct an annual evaluation to detemine the effectiveness of the program

To design a recruitment strategy for volunteers

To provide information about, and encourage access to, the adapted fitness program

Setting Behavioral or Performance Fitness Objectives for the Handicapped

Human behavior is divided into four basic learning domains: cognitive, psychomotor, affective, and psychosocial. Handicapped individuals who wish to become more competent in any of these areas need to focus on individualized goals known as "behavioral" or "performance" objectives.

To assure the reality of a behavioral objective, fitness instructors must first access the participant's overall physical and motor fitness level. Thereafter, the instructor devises a program that estimates the probability of the participant's reaching a certain level of fitness within a designated time, space, or both. If the participant fails to meet these requirements, the question should be asked, "What kind of instruction, and how much, is needed to gain a reasonable level of fitness?" It is possible for the instructor to observe a disabled person's response to tests and to measure, record, and evaluate them. A trainable mentally retarded with poor cardiovascular endurance, may, for example, swim the width of the pool three out of five trials, a performance that fulfills a behavioral objective according to five criteria:

The Situation

The name, background, handicapping condition, and present physical fitness level of the participant or student.

The Movement

The fitness activities concerned with cardiovascular endurance, muscular strength, muscular endurance, flexibility, or combinations of these.

The Condition

The term refers here to everything of an auxiliary or facilitating nature, from prosthetic devices to direct physical aid by the instructor to no assistance at all.

The Challenge

Stipulations relating to the amount of space and time involved in performing a fitness activity. Thus, a handicapped person may be "challenged" to jog several blocks or half a mile in half an hour, more or less.

Degree of Achievement

The instructor and the participant may both ask to what extent the "challenge" has been met in accordance with the prescribed device or aid.

These five criteria are only practical steps toward the fulfillment of behavioral objectives and should not be used without several cautionary remarks. First of all, administrators and instructors should agree on the relevance and appropriateness of the objectives. Second, these objectives must be capable of duplication. When other fitness instructors may wish to offer similar or identical fitness activities to their participants, the criteria above should be available. Third, not only the ends but also the means must be scrutinized. Everything considered leading or teaching — methods, techniques facilities, equipment, supplies — should be consistent with the end in view. That end is a measurable achievement.

The following examples illustrate a method for preparing and recording behavioral objectives. In each case, the first criterion ("situation") should be more detailed regarding home situation, body image, weight, and both physical and emotional readiness:

Situation: Jane, a fourteen-year-old with Down's Syndrome.
Movement: Jogging (fast pace).
Condition: Unassisted.
Challenge: One mile in fourteen minutes.

Degree of Achievement: Having succeeded in covering the distance in fourteen minutes and forty seconds, she performed successfully and was advised to go into a weight-training program but still continue jogging.

Situation: Joe, a twenty-four-year-old with cerebral palsy.
Movement: Walking ("as best you can").
Condition: With braces, but unassisted.
Challenge: Without stopping, walk along a straight plastic tape fifty feet in length placed on sidewalk.
Degree of Achievement: Joe did wobble in his braces, but his diligence and perseverance earned him recognition for a successful performance.

Even at a brief glance, these examples will indicate the central importance of behavioral objectives. Instructors should clearly understand how each objective is developed and how it relates to the participant in question. Each articulates the "What," "Why" and "How" of the participant's physical and motor fitness level. Finally, each objective, once recorded, provides instructors with a measurable account of progress and participants with some degree of achievement.

RELATIONSHIP OF FITNESS GOALS TO FITNESS OBJECTIVES IN THE INDIVIDUALIZED EDUCATION PROGRAM

Among several key provisions in the Education for All Handicapped Children Act, Public Law 94-142, is the stipulation that as part of a free appropriate education guaranteed every handicapped child, an individualized education program must be developed and implemented for **every** child receiving special education and related services. Since instruction in physical education is a defined part of special education under P.L. 94-142, it is logical that physical education should be part of the individualized education program for every handicapped child receiving special education and related services.

Having given a brief background on the Individualized Education Program, our major concern now is the relationship of fitness goals to fitness objectives. As individualized education programs are approached for any given number of participants or students, a number of factors must be considered if fitness activities are to result in fulfillment of meaningful goals and relevant objectives for a particular student. The following questions must be answered before any decisions are made:

- Are the goals appropriate for that student?
- Are the objectives relevant for that student?
- Is the student's handicapping condition taken into account?
- Are the student's present physical and motor fitness levels considered?
- Are there sequences and progressions for the fitness activity to be taught?
- Are the instructional methods and techniques to be used familiar to the instructor?
- Will the student be in the "least restrictive environment" to maximize learning?
- What fitness adaptations or accommodations will be necessary?
- How many and what types of fitness tests will be used to determine the student's needs?

In conclusion, a "goal" usually refers to a higher level of competence in any one of a number of fitness activities, games, or sports. In an Individualized Education Program (IEP), neither the number or complexity of the activities or sports that comprise a "goal" is fixed; specifications are always relative to the student's needs and are never absolute. Objectives, on the other hand, can be reached as interim check points indicating the student's progress. The immediate advantage of such a "pacer" is that it discourages slow-downs and reduces needless deviations. It also provides frequent rewards for even the most modest signs of progress. Thus, it is important that accurate records be kept on each student who participates.

Chapter V

PLANNING AND ORGANIZING FITNESS CLASSES AND PROGRAMS

SINCE a good environment is essential for effective teaching or leading, the teacher or leader must plan and organize the classes and programs. Although physical fitness by its very nature is conducted in a relaxed atmosphere, still the instruction must be carried on in an orderly fashion. A number of important factors are involved in planning and organizing fitness classes and programs.

GROUPINGS FOR FITNESS CLASSES

Should fitness classes be grouped according to chronological age, mental age, physical size, kind of handicap, degree of handicap, physical fitness level, or general motor fitness? No formula exists that will provide an appropriate answer. Much depends on the considerations above and on the number of participants involved and the instructor-participant ratio. Of major importance is the fact that all class members participate in a fitness program.

Groupings which promote various dimensions of physical fitness among the handicapped must be carefully designed to meet the needs and the capacities of all participants. Consideration must be given to the aspects of fitness desired — cardiovascular endurance (aerobic capacity), muscular strength, muscular endurance, flexibility, or a combination of these.

In schools, the most logical place to conduct physical fitness activities is in physical education classes. Here fitness can be integrated with the teaching of gross-motor and game-and-sports skills. This type of placement should work well in both the mainstream and the adapted programs. A problem will arise when physical education classes are taught by elementary classroom teachers who do not have the background to teach physical fitness activities. For those teachers having in-service training, studying the literature will be helpful as well as other learning opportunities.

Fitness may also be taught in the health education curriculum. The integration of physical fitness into the health education area has merit: Students receive knowledge based on all aspects of health in the health education classes and perform the practical work in fitness in physical education classes. Although some handicapped students may not comprehend health education subject-matter, they can still participate in fitness activities.

Regardless of how disabled students are grouped, instruction in physical fitness can still be effective; the key is the effectiveness of the teacher.

CLASS SIZE AND COMPOSITION

The physical fitness class size and composition will depend upon answers to the following questions:

- How many days a week are physical fitness classes offered?
- If integrated with physical education, what percentage of time is devoted to physical fitness?
- What is the time allotment for physical fitness?
- Are adequate facilities and equipment available?
- Is the fitness class mainstreamed or adapted?
- Are the teachers trained to teach fitness activities to the handicapped?

When handicapped students are placed in a mainstreamed class for physical fitness activities, there is no ready-made formula that dictates the cutoff point for class size. Each class has its own particular problems. Usually, a ratio of six to eight regular students to each handicapped student in a class of 20 to 25 is considered manageable.

However, if the total enrollment is unmanageable, the number of handicapped should be reduced. Mental age, chronological age, physical fitness level, motor efficiency, cognitive skill, and both so-cial and emotional stability all figure in decisions on class size and composition.

Adapted fitness classes are seldom homogenous with respect to physical, mental, social, emotional or functional handicaps or any combinations of these. Each handicapped student's needs, interests, and potential must be recognized before he/she can build upon abili-ties and reduce deficiencies. As homogeneity is usually lacking in an adapted class, the instructor is expected to accommodate each stu-dent.

Adapted classes in which fitness is taught usually have an en-rollment that ranges from 8 to 15 students. The kind and degree of handicapping condition, the present physical condition of the student, the instructor's background, and the facilities and equipment available all affect decisions on class size and composi-tion.

When physical fitness classes are conducted in non-school set-tings, no formula exists to determine class size and composition. Factors that must be considered are the same as for schools; but there is, however, more homogeneity in some non-school than in school settings. For example, in institutions for the men-tally retarded or in schools for the deaf or the blind, participants can very well be taught fitness activities in classes of 15 to 20 individ-uals.

FORMATIONS USED TO PRESENT
EXERCISES AND FITNESS ACTIVITIES

In many cases much instructional time is lost in selecting the ap-propriate formation(s) that should be used in fitness classes. It is im-portant that participants have specific positions in reference to one another and to the instructor. Formations that are described here in-clude circle, semi-circle, line, relay, couple or small group, and spread.

To assist with individual placements in formations, the instructor may use colored masking tape or tape inscribed with the participant's name stuck to the floor at prearranged locations to designate the place where the instructor wants that individual to stand, sit, or lie or where he/she wants the wheelchair to be located. In the following diagrams, the position of the instructor is indicated by an "I" and the position of the participant by an "X."

Circle Formation

All participants join hands. The instructor takes the hand of the first individual and leads the group around into a circle formation. The instructor remains an integral part of the circle and remains either inside or outside. The instructor must be seen and heard by everyone. This formation may be used for all locomotion movements.

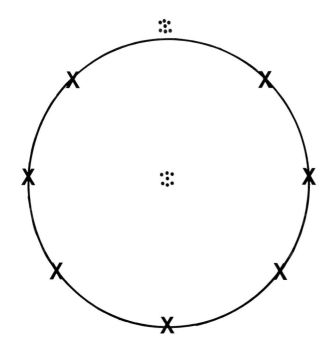

Semi-Circle Formation

Participants should be spaced off to allow for calisthenics, jump rope, running in place, or relaxation exercises.

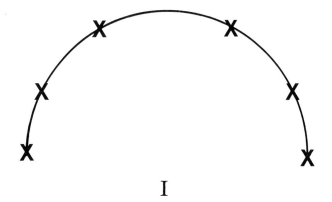

I

Line Formation

This formation may be used for marching, calisthenics, jump rope, running in place, or locomotor movements. It may also be used for sprints/dashes.

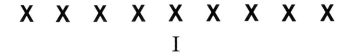

I

Relay Formation

This formation may be used for all types of locomotor relays with or without equipment. It may also be used for couple or small-group activities and for assisted exercises, isometrics, and weight-training with barbells and dumbbells.

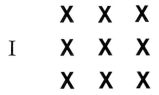

Spread Formation

Participants select a spot at random but must allow enough space from one another for performing exercises and fitness activities.

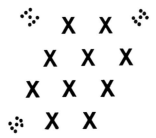

TIME ALLOTMENT

The amount of time devoted to the teaching or leading of physical fitness activities depends upon several factors. The philosophy of the establishment, type of program presently offered, ages, handicapping conditions, functioning level of the participants, the instructor's training and background, and the facilities and equipment available — all of these factors must again be considered.

In schools, adapted physical education classes should meet once a day from 20 to 25 minutes depending on the students involved. It is recommended that at least 25 percent of the time be devoted to the teaching of fitness activities, and in many cases more time should be allocated. There may be modules in which all of the class time is spent on physical fitness activities. Furthermore, the whole physical education program could very well be called the physical and motor fitness program whereby the teaching of basic motor skills is incorporated into the teaching of fitness activities.

In institutions and recreation department settings, physical activity programs may be conducted only once or twice a week. These sessions usually range from one to one-and-a-half hours. In general, these types of programs consist of recreational sports intermixed with physical fitness activities. The recent trend, however, calls for more time to be allocated to fitness programs and activities than is presently being given.

In hospital rehabilitation departments, patients should spend at least thirty minutes a day working on a progressive resistance weight program. Here the limiting factors may be too many patients, not enough physical therapists, and lack of facilities and equipment. If daily workouts are not possible, forty-five minute sessions every other day will suffice.

FITNESS PROGRAM CONTRACTS

When students reach a decision that they are prepared to participate in a fitness program, the agreement between the participants and the instructor is a bond and is called a "contract." Whenever possible, the handicapped student should fill out the contract; subsequently it must be approved by the instructor. Once the fitness program is implemented, any changes necessary must have instructor approval. The instructor must monitor the participant's progress on a weekly basis. When the participant has completed the fitness program, the instructor signs the contract. If, however, the program is not completed, the instructor must indicate on the contract the reason(s) for its termination.

FACILITIES

Most administration books on health, physical education, and recreation devote at least one chapter to facilities for the regular population. But within the last ten years, because of federal and state laws, both indoor and outdoor facilities for the handicapped have received a great deal of attention. There are those who recommend that the same facilities be used by everyone — a very commendable recommendation. But people who make this recommendation do not know, nor do they understand, the needs of the disabled population.

Before any decision can be made as to what constitutes adequate fitness facilities for the handicapped two important questions must be answered: What are the kinds and degrees of handicapping conditions? What are the actual and potential physical and motor fitness abilities of the handicapped users? The key to any kinds of facilities for the disabled population is accessibility.

Perhaps the best approach for fitness programmers to determine facility utilization by the handicapped is to be aware of the following considerations:

Indoor Facilities

- Is there a ramp which leads into the facility?
- Are the corridors wide enough to accommodate wheelchairs?

- Are the floors safe for those on crutches as well as those with braces?
- Is the facility floor free from dust?
- Is the air temperature in the facility controlled?
- Can the facility accommodate walking or jogging classes?
- Are there signs and markings either in Braille or in raised letters?
- Are the aisles in the locker rooms of the non-skid type?
- Are some of the toilets in the locker rooms designed to accommodate wheelchairs?
- Are some of the hand lavatories, mirrors, towel racks and drinking fountains at the proper heights to accommodate those in wheelchairs?
- Are some of the showers designed for wheelchair participants?
- Are audio-cassettes or other sound-warnings installed for the visually impaired?

Indoor Swimming Pools

- Is there adequate lighting?
- Is there adequate deck space around the pool?
- Are the deck floors made of non-skid materials?
- Is there a ramp that leads into the pool?
- Is there a lift in the pool?
- Is there proper water temperature control?
- Do the overflow gutters function properly?
- Is there a shallow end in the pool?
- Is there enough room in the pool to play water games?
- Is there enough room in the pool for the use of equipment?
- Is there proper mechanical ventilation in the pool?
- Is there adequate acoustical treatment of walls and ceilings?

Outdoor Facilities

- Is there a bike path available?
- Is there a par course designed to accommodate wheelchairs?
- Is there a walking or jogging course designed to accommodate wheelchairs?
- Is there an annual wheelchair marathon race?

- Is the outdoor pool accessible to the handicapped?
- Is there a lake, pond, or ocean that is accessible to the handicapped?
- Are the winter sports facilities accessible to the disabled?
- Are the community's fitness and sports facilities accessible to the disabled?

EQUIPMENT

The term "equipment," as used in this text, refers to non-expendable items. These have longevity, needing only occasional repair or replacement. A few examples of fitness equipment are skinfold calipers, stationary bicycles, and weight-training machines. The kinds and numbers of pieces of equipment needed will vary according to the situation. For example, a hospital rehabilitation department would not have a weight-training machine, whereas a school would find such a piece of equipment most useful.

For the purpose of this discussion, two kinds of equipment are identified — testing, and workout or training equipment. However, some testing equipment can also be used for conditioning purposes. It must be pointed out again, however, that each type of fitness program will dictate equipment needs. Of course, finances available for the program will be a determining factor.

The following pieces of equipment are listed under each category mentioned above:

Testing Equipment

Arm Ergometer	Sit and Reach Apparatus
Bench Press	Skinfold Calipers
Bicycle Ergometer	Sphygmomanometer
Flexometer	Stethoscope
Goniometer	Timer
Hand Dynometer	Tracer
Leg Press	*Treadmill
Mat	Twelve Inch Thigh Bench

---

*Optional; if purchased, recorders are necessary.

Metronome

Scale with Height Indicator

Vitalograph spirometer or regular spirometer

Yardstick

Workout, or Training, Equipment

Air Flow Mat(s)

Ankle Weights

Arm Wheel

Barbells

Barrels

Bench(s)

Climbing Rope(s)

Collars

Dumbbells

Elastic Cables

Foam Wedge Mat

Full Body Suspension Walker

Inclined Walker

Ladder

Leather Belt(s) (for lower backs)

Logs

Mat(s) (regular)

Mini-Gym Isokinetic Apparatus

Mini Trampoline(s)

Mirror(s)

Musical Equipment — tapes/records

Nautilus Sports Machines

Parachute

Plowing Machine

Portable Treadmill

Scooter Boards

Springs

Stair Platform with Rails

Stall Bars

Stationary Bicycle(s)

Tricycle(s)

Tunnel(s)

Universal Gym Equipment

Up-and-Down Ramp

Walker on Wheels or Roller Walker

Weighted Plates

Whiz Wheel

Wrist Weights

SUPPLIES

The term "supplies" is interpreted as expendable items. These must be replaced over a relatively short period of time. A few examples are wands, hoops, and jump ropes. The following list of supplies should suffice for most adapted fitness programs:

Balloons

Basketballs

Medicine Ball

Nerf Balls, audible

Beanbags
Cageball
Chalk — Carbonate of
  Magnesia
Dowels
Electronic Balls with
  Beepers
Flagbelts
Footballs
Hoops, plastic
Individual Jump Ropes
Masking Tape
Measuring Tape
Paddles with elastic
  attachments to balls
Plastic Tape
Playground Balls, assorted
  sizes
Roller Skates
Rubber Inner Tubes (assorted)
Rubber Rings
Soccer Balls
Sponge Balls
Stop Watch
Traffic Cone Markers

SAFETY MEASURES

Precautions must be taken to reduce the chance of injury to participants in fitness programs. The elimination of hazards in instruction, facilities, and equipment is extremely important. Fitness instructors should regularly question their own teaching and constantly point out hazards to their participants.

The following safety measures should prove helpful and are listed under the topics of instruction, equipment, and facilities.

Instruction

- Medical examination must be required of all participants.
- Fitness classes should never be unsupervised.
- Trained and qualified instructors are a must.
- Spotters must be utilized whenever necessary.
- Proper instruction must precede performance for any type of fitness activity.
- Proper instruction is essential for using fitness machines and equipment.
- Instructors must stress warm-ups to avoid injury to muscles, joints or ligaments.
- Instructors should not allow participants to lift an excessive amount of weights that may cause strain.

- Rhythmic breathing is recommended while weight-training.
- Hands should be free from perspiration while weight-training.
- Instructors should emphasize correct body positions for weight-training.
- The instructor should know how and when to spot fatigue.
- Instructors should watch carefully participants who are subject to seizures.
- Instructors should stop the activity if the participant complains of pain to any part of the body, has dyspnea (shortness of breath), has abnormal coloring of the face, feels fatigue, or has cyanosis (blueness of the lips).
- Instructors should allow frequent rest periods for participants with heart problems.
- Instructors should be certified in C.P.R.
- Instructors should stress cool-down periods as part of the workout.
- Instructors should know what procedures to follow in case of accidents.

Equipment

- Mats should be utilized.
- All fitness conventional equipment and machines should be inspected regularly.
- Pools should have available: safety lines, area markers, ring buoys, shepherd crooks, back boards, reaching poles and rescue tubes.
- Collars must be secured for barbell usage.
- Dumbbells should be returned to their racks after usage.
- Barbells should be returned to their racks after usage.
- Weight plates should be returned to their racks after usage.
- Knee pads should be worn for performing creeping exercises.
- Homemade equipment should be checked for safety.
- Par course exercise stations should be inspected regularly.

Facilities

- Floors of locker and shower rooms should be of non-skid type.
- Deck floors of pools should be of non-skid type.

- Pool lifts should be inspected regularly.
- Sufficient space should be allowed between each exercise station.
- Participants with balance difficulties or frail bones should be assisted in walking on wet floors and ramps.
- Rails should be inspected regularly.
- Ramps should be inspected regularly.
- Corridors should be inspected regularly for broken tiles.
- Exercise area floors should be inspected regularly.
- Exercise areas should be dust free.

Chapter VI

ASSESSING PARTICIPANTS
FOR PROGRAM PLACEMENT

ASSESSMENT, as used in this text, is a process whereby the results of tests are used to evaluate the individual and are interpreted as bases for decision-making relative to program planning and placement. Before any fitness test is administered, the most important evaluation is the medical examination. This comprehensive examination will provide a means for the discovery of any defects or problems the participant may have and also can help to determine the individual's entry level into a fitness program.

Assessing participants accurately for entry into fitness programs is most crucial. Therefore, it is recommended that only specific and objective type tests be administered. Tests selected should provide uniformity of scoring, consistent measuring, and overall ease of administering. Additionally, time and equipment required to perform the tests should be minimal. Norm tables on some tests are always appropriate to use. Conversely, the instructor may wish to use the self-testing approach whereby participants' scores are compared against themselves. This type of evaluation can readily reveal if they have improved or progressed to any degree.

Although standing height and weight measurements are included in the medical examination, they should also be taken as part of any physical fitness test. These types of measurements should also be included in the exercise prescription. Only after test results are interpreted and analyzed can accurate exercise prescriptions be formulated. In addition, resting heart rate and resting blood pressure measurements are part of the assessment.

Other measurements which can prove helpful if the disabled person is to be placed in an isotonic or weight training program are body measurements. A cloth tape measure is used, and measurements are recorded in inches to the nearest quarter of an inch.

Body measurements should include: chest-normal, flexed (male), bustline (female); midriff (female); upper right arm — flexed, normal; upper left arm — flexed, normal; waistline (female), waist — umbilical cord (male); hips (female); buttocks (female); upper right thigh, right calf, upper left thigh, left calf.

It must be noted that some so-called physical fitness tests include motor skill or motor fitness items. If the instructor wishes to assess specifically for physical fitness, motor skill or motor fitness items must be omitted.

A comprehensive physical fitness assessment should include five major components: muscular strength, muscular endurance, flexibility, body fat composition, and aerobic capacity. It is recommended that disabled persons who are thirty-five years of age or older and have the functional capabilities, take the "stress" test, also known as the "maximal graded exercise test" or the "aerobic capacity test." This test is based on the participants' reaching their age-predicted **maximum** heart rate. This component must be directed by a physician.

Individuals who are **under** thirty-five years of age and have the functional capabilities take the "stress" test known as the "**submaximal** graded exercise test" or "aerobic capacity test." This test is based on the participants' reaching 75-85 percent of their age-predicted maximum heart rate. This type of aerobic capacity assessment does not require the presence of a physician but does require that the tester be trained in testing protocol.

TESTING PRELIMINARIES

Following are the testing procedures to be used for a comprehensive physical fitness assessment.* It should be administered in the

---

*These assessment procedures were designed for the regular population; however, they may be adapted to serve disabled individuals.

order as indicated below. Only the first four components — muscular strength, muscular endurance, flexibility and body fat composition — should be tested at one session. Aerobic capacity should be tested at another session.*

Standing Height

Facing the height indicator, the individual should stand barefooted on a scale, heels together, arms at the sides, and body fully extended. Heels, buttocks, upper back, and head are in a straight line. The chin must be kept in a level position. Measurement is recorded in inches to the nearest quarter of an inch.

Weight

The individual should wear shorts, T-shirt, and no shoes. Record weight in pounds to the nearest quarter pound.

Resting Blood Pressure

The individual should be sitting and relaxed. Measurement is taken in the artery of the upper arm with a sphygmomanometer. The rubber cuff is wrapped around the arm and air is pumped into the cuff by a rubber bulb. A stethoscope is placed over the artery and the air pressure is slowly released. Tapping sounds are heard as the blood begins to flow. The first tapping sound heard is the **systolic** pressure, when the heart is contracting. A point is reached when the tapping sounds change suddenly to very soft sounds and then disappear entirely. The point at which the sound disappears is the **diastolic** pressure, when the heart is resting. The measures are usually written 120/80. The top number is systolic; the bottom number is diastolic.

Resting Heart Rate

The individual feels the pulse by placing two or three fingers lightly on the inside of the wrist with the thumb on the top of the wrist. The thumb is never used to take a pulse reading because the

---

*Norm tables for the comprehensive physical fitness assessment for the regular population may be found in Kenneth H. Cooper, *The Aerobics Program for Total Well-Being* and in *Health and Fitness Through Physical Activity* by Michael L. Pollock, Jack H. Wilmore and Samuel M. Fox III.

thumb has its own pulse. The number of beats per minute is the pulse rate.

TESTS AND PROCEDURES

The following tests and procedures are essential for a comprehensive physical fitness assessment:

Muscular Strength

Authorities recommend that muscle strength be assessed by having the disabled person lift a maximum load once or one repetition (1RM). A major muscle or muscle group must be selected. The test is administered through a series of trial and error lifts. That is, start with a weight the handicapped person can lift; then keep adding weights until a weight is found that can be lifted comfortably, without strain or pain. The individual being tested should learn to exhale while he/she lifts the weight.

In this text, two tests that determine muscle strength will be described, the seated leg press and the supine bench press. Some handicapped individuals, because of their functional capabilities, will not be able to be tested for muscle strength.

Seated Leg Press

The individual sits on the seat of a weight training machine and places the feet on the lifting levers. Hips must be pressed firmly against the seat and the seat should be adjusted so that the knees and hips are flexed at least 90 degrees. The lifting levers are pressed forward until the legs are fully extended, then returned slowly to the starting position.

Bench Press

The individual lies in supine position on the bench under the lifting lever of a weight training machine so that the lifting lever is in line with the upper chest. The lifting lever is pressed upward to full-arm extension and lowered slowly to starting position until the weights on the lifting lever touch the weights on the stack. The head, shoulders, and buttocks should remain in contact with the bench throughout the press.

Muscular Endurance

Since any test used to measure muscular endurance will be subjective, this component will be difficult to assess because of the number of different muscles and muscle groups in the body. Experts in the field of physical fitness recommend that the push-up and timed sit-up tests be used to measure upper body and abdominal muscular strength. A word of caution — both of these tests are greatly dependent on the participant's motivation.

Push-ups

Dependent upon male or female and the type of disability, both the full and modified push-up may be utilized. For the full push-ups, the individual assumes a prone rest start position with the head, back, hips and legs in a straight line. In the starting position, the arms are fully extended and toes are on the floor to support the body. The chest is slowly lowered by bending the arms so that the chest lightly touches the floor, then returns to the starting position. The body must remain straight throughout the test. The number of correctly performed push-ups is recorded.

Modified Push-ups

For the modified push-ups, the individual assumes a prone rest start position with the arms fully extended and knees bent resting on the mat, as the heels of the feet are pointed toward the head. The chest is slowly lowered by bending the arms so that the chest lightly touches the mat, then returns to the starting position. An alternate method is for the individual to perform this test utilizing a 12-inch bench or a lower run of bleachers for front support of the arms, the body fully extended, with the toes touching the floor. The number of correctly performed push-ups is recorded.

Timed Sit-ups

The individual assumes a supine position on a mat with the fingers lightly grasping the head, covering the ears. Knees are bent, feet flat on the mat and slightly apart. The instructor must hold down both ankles. The back is curled up and the trunk is raised until the trunk is vertical to the floor and both elbows touch the thighs. The individual returns to the starting position and repeats the movement. The instructor counts the number of sit-ups performed correctly in either thirty or sixty seconds depending on the person's physical capacity.

Flexibility

The best way to assess flexibility of various joints is by using the Leighton Flexometer and the electrogniometer. However, in many situations these pieces of equipment may not be available. Therefore, the sit and reach or the standard reach tests are good substitutes. Either of these tests measures the flexibility of the posterior leg muscles and the lower back, a good indication of a person's body flexibility.

Sit and Reach

The individual assumes a sitting position with knees fully extended and the soles of the feet against a box, board or bench. The hands and arms are stretched forward by bending the trunk, and this position is held for three seconds. The knees must remain extended. A ruler or yardstick is used to measure the distance in front of, or beyond, the edge of the bench, and the distance is recorded in inches to the nearest quarter of an inch.

Stand and Reach

The individual stands close to the edge of a 12-inch high bench and slowly bends downward to determine how far down he/she can reach. Knees must be held straight. The instructor holds a yardstick at the edge of the bench and records the distance from the floor to the tips of the fingers in inches to the nearest quarter of an inch.

Body Fat Composition

The most appropriate way to measure body fat is by the use of skinfold calipers. The Lange or the Harpenden are most commonly used; moreover, the measurements become more reliable and valid with the instructor's practice. Both of these calipers are designed to measure the fat that lies directly beneath the skin, or the subcutaneous fat. Regardless of how far apart the caliper jaws spread, the tension between the jaws remains constant. Measurements are taken from the right side of the body and recorded in millimeters by someone other than the instructor.

- Grasp the skinfold between the thumb and forefinger. The skinfold should be grasped several times and then held to make certain that the skinfold does not include muscle.
- Place the calipers on the fold one centimeter below the fingers and release the fingers slightly so that the pressure is on the caliper, not on the fingers.
- The individual is standing and each fold is taken in a vertical plane except for the subscapular, which is measured on a slight slant in a lateral plane in the natural fold of the skin.
- When the movement of the needle stops, take the reading to the nearest half millimeter.
- Three readings should be taken at each site and the average recorded.
- The four anatomical sites for skinfold are triceps, suprailiac, thigh, and subscapula.

Stress (Cardiovascular Endurance) (Aerobic Capacity) Assessment*

The preparation portion may be done in two ways, with skin electrodes or an electrode belt. The belt is simply secured around the participant's chest, the metal electrodes in good contact with the skin. This method may be unreliable during peak exercise because of exaggerated electrode movement.

In addition to the belt, skin electrodes are used. They provide a secure contact and are accurate measurements of the heart rate. The three skin sites must first be rubbed with gauze pads and alcohol to remove oil and dirt, after which a pumice-like jelly is applied to further reduce resistance and insure a more accurate signal.

---

*If the reader wishes more detailed information on cardiovascular endurance or aerobic capacity testing, refer to American College of Sports Medicine, *Guidelines for Graded Exercise Testing and Exercise Prescription* and The Committee on Exercise, Albert A. Kattus, Chairman, *Exercise Testing and Training of Apparently Healthy Individuals: A Handbook for Physicians.*

Selection of skin sites is generally in the form of a triangle, one located under the right collarbone and two spread apart under the lower ribs. The type of selection provides what is commonly known as a "Lead II" rhythm strip for heart rate monitoring. When the electrodes are in position on the skin sites, they should be secured with an ace bandage.

In a laboratory setting, aerobic capacity can be determined in three ways: by use of a treadmill, a bicycle ergometer, or an arm ergometer. Additionally, a simple step test or a 1.5 mile run/walk will also provide the instructor with data that may be used to determine cardiovascular endurance. The resting heart rate is taken and recorded before the participant begins the actual test. Vital signs are recorded at the end of each stage (stages vary from two to three minutes' duration) of the selected procedures until the participant reaches 85 percent of his/her maximum age-predicted heart rate. At this point, the participant begins recovery. Vital signs are recorded at two minute intervals until the resting values are reached.

If the test has gone well and there has been no abnormal response — fatigue, light headedness, shortness of breath — and the participant had a steady and appropriate blood pressure response, an exercise prescription may be written. The prescription is based on using 75 percent to 85 percent of the maximum age-predicted heart rate for exercise. Norms developed by Cooper are available; and by using these, the participant may be placed into a category of aerobic fitness, that is, either low, average, or high.

Other Tests to Determine
Aerobic Capacity

There are three simple tests which have been widely accepted to measure cardiovascular endurance (aerobic capacity). These tests may be utilized when mass testing is desired and they also may serve as self-tests. They require minimal equipment to administer and have been proven to be almost as accurate and reliable as laboratory tests. Again, with the disabled population, motivation will be the key.

Three-Minute Step Test

The individual steps up and down upon a bench which is approximately 12-16 inches high. The lower row of bleachers is usually satisfactory for this test. The step up and down is counted as one repetition and is continued for three minutes. A metronome should be used. Upon completion of the test, the individual remains standing while the pulse is counted for 60 seconds beginning 5 seconds after the test has terminated.

Twelve-Minute Test

Each individual attempts to run and walk as far as possible, maintaining a comfortable pace for twelve minutes. If the individual gets winded, he/she may slow down to a walk until the breath is recovered; then he/she continues to run. This procedure can be used throughout the test. The measurement for this test is the greatest distance covered in twelve minutes.

1.5 Mile Test

This simple test is a modification of the 12-minute test mentioned above. It is usually used for large group testing. The test, which is based on the time required to run 1.5 miles, is easy to administer and to interpret.

Vital Lung Capacity Assessment

An optional test which may be used in a comprehensive physical fitness assessment is called vital lung capacity. If a vitalograph spirometer or a less sophisticated spirometer is available, this test may be administered. This test may prove helpful in evaluating the lung volume of handicapped persons.

The procedure used in spirometry testing is as follows:

The spirometer is set and the mouthpiece is attached. The individual should be standing in an erect position. The mouthpiece is inserted into the individual's mouth and must be held firmly between the teeth and lips but not bitten. The instructor then tells the individual to take as deep a breath as possible (aspiration). Upon the request "blow out" (expiration), the participant expels all the air as rapidly and completely as possible without stopping. (The instructor should demonstrate the proper technique of inhaling and exhaling before the actual test begins).

When the individual is ready, the instructor starts the spirometer and tells the individual to take a very deep breath and then blow it out. The instructor should watch for nose and mouth leaks as well as bends or dents in the mouthpiece or tubing. The individual should be encouraged to perform complete inhales as the instructor says, "Keep exhaling," "keep exhaling."

One practice trial is allowed before the two tests for which the results are recorded. The measurements are taken in liters. The value of forced vital capacity (FVC) depends on the person's age, sex, and height.

The spirometer standards for normal males and females may be determined by using a nomogram published by the American Thoracic Society, Medical Section of the American Lung Association, 1740 Broadway, New York, New York, 10019.

STANDARDIZED TESTS SPECIFICALLY DESIGNED FOR THE HANDICAPPED

Several standardized physical fitness tests designed for the handicapped are now available. Some of these tests measure only physical fitness, but in some cases they will include motor fitness items. As one examines each test battery, tests which include motor fitness items can readily be detected. Information as to the source of these instruments and the population they serve will be noted in alphabetical order. Each instrument will indicate what is assessed and/or the test items.

BUELL ADAPTATION OF THE AAHPER YOUTH FITNESS TEST FOR THE BLIND AND PARTIALLY SEEING

Population served: Visually handicapped youngsters aged 10-17.

Components	Test Items
Speed	50-yard dash
Arm and shoulder girdle strength	Pull-ups (boys)
	Knee push-ups (girls)

Abdominal and hip strength	Sit-ups (bent legs)
Leg strength and power	Standing broad jump
Cardiovascular endurance	600-yard run-walk
Body agility and coordination	Squat thrusts (10 seconds)
Arm strength and coordination	Basketball throw

Sources: The publication, *Physical Education and Recreation for the Visually Handicapped*, which includes all the norms and details of tests, is available from American Alliance Publications, P.O. Box 704, Waldorf, Maryland 20601. Write for purchase information or order by phone: (703) 476-3481. In addition, refer to Charles E. Buell, *Physical Education For Blind Children*, 2nd ed., 1983, Courtesy of Charles C Thomas, Publisher, Springfield, Illinois.

MOTOR FITNESS TESTING MANUAL FOR THE MODERATELY MENTALLY RETARDED

Population served: Moderately mentally retarded boys and girls, aged 6-21.

What Is Measured	**Test Items**
Arm and shoulder girdle strength	Flexed-arm hang
Abdominal and hip strength	Sit-ups (30 seconds)
Leg strength and power	Standing long jump
Arm strength and coordination	Softball throw for distance
Speed	50-yard dash
Cardiovascular endurance	300-yard run-walk
Flexibility	Sitting bob-and-reach
Development skills	Motor fitness related:
	Hopping
	Skipping
	Tumbling progression
	Target throw

Source: The publication, *Motor Fitness Testing for the Moderately Mentally Retarded*, which includes all the norms and details of tests, is available from American Alliance Publications, P.O. Box 704,

Waldorf, Maryland 20601. Write for purchase information or order by phone: (703) 476-3481.

PHYSICAL FITNESS TEST FOR THE TRAINABLE MENTALLY RETARDED

Population served: Mentally retarded boys and girls, aged 8-17.

What Is Measured	Test Items
Arm and shoulders	Hang for time
	Medicine ball throw
Back	Back extension flexibility
	Speed back lifts (30 seconds)
Abdomen	Speed sit-ups (30 seconds)
Legs	Vertical jump
	Floor touch flexibility
Organic fitness	300-yard run

Source: Frank J. Hayden, *Physical Fitness for the Mentally Retarded.* Toronto: 1964, 48 pp. (Contact: School of Physical Education and Athletics, McMaster University, Hamiltion, Ontario, Canada).

Norms: The norms are available from the source.

PROJECT "ACTIVE"

This project includes both motor ability and physical fitness tests. However, for the purpose of this text, only the physical fitness tests will be listed.

Population served: normal, emotionally disturbed, mentally retarded, and learning disabled individuals, grades K-12.

Physical Fitness Test: (This test should be used as a
Level I   screening device.)

Factors	Test Items
Arm and shoulder strength	Static arm hang

Abdominal strength   Modified sit-ups
Explosive leg power   Standing broad jump
Cardiorespiratory endurance Running

Physical Fitness Test:
Level II

Arm and shoulder strength Static arm hang
Abdominal strength   Modified sit-ups
Explosive leg power   Standing broad jump
Cardiorespiratory endurance 200-yard dash, ages 6-11
            (grades 1-6)
            8-minute run, ages 12-13
            (grades 7-8)
            12-minute run, ages 14-18
            (grades 9-12)

Source: Thomas M. Vodola, Director, Project A.C.T.I.V.E., Township of Ocean School District, 163 Monmouth Road, Oakhurst, New Jersey 07755, (1978).

Norms: The norms are available from the author. (VEE, Inc., P.O. Box 2093, Neptune City, New Jersey 07753).

PROJECT "I CAN"

Population served: Severely handicapped individuals, aged 4-25.

There are 8 instructional modules, 4 primary level and 4 secondary level; however, the focus of this text is on physical fitness, so only the Fitness and Growth Module is considered.

What Is Measured

Abdominal strength
Arm/Shoulder strength
Heart/Lung strength
Trunk/Leg flexibility

Source: Hubbard, P.O. Box 104, Northbrook, Illinois 60062. Michigan State University, East Lansing, Michigan 48823 (1976).

Norms: The norms are available from the source.

PROJECT "UNIQUE"

Population served: Sensory and orthopedically impaired children and youth, aged 10-17.

Project Unique Physical Fitness Test Items X Major Subject Groups

Subject Group	Test Items*
Normal, Auditory Impaired, and Visually Impaired Boys and Girls	**Basic Test**: Body composition: triceps skinfold, subscapular skinfold, sum of triceps and subscapula skinfolds; strength: right grip, left grip, sum of grips; power-speed: 50-yard/meter dash; power strength: sit-ups; flexibility: sit and reach; cardiorespiratory endurance: long distance run. **Substitions**: The broad jump may be substituted for grip strength tests as a measure of strength.
Cerebral Palsy	**Basic Test**: The basic test includes the same items as recommended for normal individuals except that the sit-up test is eliminated and girls substitute the softball throw for distance as a measure of power-strength. The 50-yard/meter dash is a measure of power-endurance. In the case of cerebral palsy boys, grip tests are measures of power-strength. **Substitutions**: The arm hang may be substituted for grip tests as measures of power-strength for boys.
Paraplegic Wheelchair Spinal Neuromuscular	**Basic Test**: The basic test includes the same items as recommended for normal individuals except that the sit-up and sit and reach tests are eliminated. The 50-yard/meter dash is used as a measure of power-endurance. **Substitutions**: The arm hang or softball throw for distance may be substituted for grip strength measures (strength factor) for male subjects. The softball throw may be substituted

Congenital Anomaly/Amputee

for grip strength measures (strength factor) for female subjects.

Basic Test: The basic test items for this group are the same as for normal subjects.

Substitutions: As a substitute for grip tests, boys may substitute the broad jump or arm hang and girls may substitute the broad jump as measures of the strength factor, as appropriate. The softball throw for distance may be substituted for sit-ups (as a power-strength factor) in cases when the sit-up would be considered inappropriate.

*In certain cases, test items may be modified for particular groups and be eliminated for subgroups within groups when the administration of a particular test item would be inappropriate.

Source: Joseph P. Winnick and Francis X. Short. *The Physical Fitness of Sensory and Orthopedically Impaired Youth.* Project UNIQUE Final Report, 629 pages, November, 1982, Physical Education Department, State University of New York, College at Brockport, Brockport, New York 14420.

Project Unique Physical Fitness Test for Normal, Sensory Impaired, and Orthopedically Impaired Children and Youth: Components and Test Items.

Basic Test

Component/Factor	Test Item	Comments
Body Composition	Triceps Skinfold Subscapular Skinfold Sum of Triceps and Subscapular Skinfolds	Skinfold test items are administered to all subject groups except in cases where inappropriate due to congenital anomaly or amputation.
Muscular Strength/ Endurance		
Strength or Power-Strength	Right Grip Left Grip Sum of Grips	The grip measures are administered to all subject groups except in cases where inappropriate due to physical condition. The grip tests are used as a measure of the strength

Component/Factor	Test Item	Comments
		factor in subject groups except boys with cerebral palsy. The grip tests are used as a measure of power-strength for boys with cerebral palsy.
Power-Speed or Power-Endurance	50-Yard/Meter Dash	The 50-yard/meter dash is administered to all subject groups except where inappropriate due to physical condition. Procedures for the dash are modified for certain subject groups. The dash is used as a measure of power-speed for all groups except the cerebral palsy and spinal neuromuscular groups. Relative to these groups, the dash is a measure of power-endurance.
Power-Strength	Sit-Ups	The sit-up is administered as a measure of power-strength to all major subject groups except the cerebral palsy group and spinal neuromuscular groups. In the case of individuals with congenital anomalies/amputees, it may be necessary to eliminate or modify the test for certain subgroups or substitute the softball throw for distance as a measure of power-strength.
Power-Strength	Softball Throw	The softball throw for distance is a measure of power-strength for girls with cerebral palsy and is administered, eliminated, or modified for subgroups, as appropriate.

Flexibility	Sit and Reach	The sit and reach test is administered as a measure of flexibility to normal and sensory impaired groups. It is a test item not administered to individuals with spinal neuromuscular conditions and, although administered to other orthopedically impaired groups, may require modification or elimination in certain orthopedic subgroups.
Cardiorespiratory Endurance	Long Distance Run	The long distance run is administered to all groups. In certain instances, there is a need to modify procedures.

Substitutions

Component/Factor	Test Item	Comments
Strength	Broad Jump	The broad jump is a substitute item for grip tests in the following groups: normal, auditory impaired, visually impaired, congenital anomaly/amputee (as appropriate).
Strength or Power-Strength	Arm Hang	The arm hang is a substitute test item for grip tests for boys with cerebral palsy, paraplegic wheelchair spinal neuromuscular boys, and boys classified as congenital anomaly/amputee (as appropriate). In the case of boys with cerebral palsy, the arm hang is a measure of power-strength.
Strength or Power-Strength	Softball Throw for Distance	The softball throw for distance may be substituted as a measure of power-strength for individuals

Component/Factor	Test Item	Comments
		classified as congenital anomaly/amputee. It is used as a substitute measure of strength in the case of paraplegic wheelchair spinal neuromuscular subjects.

SPECIAL FITNESS TEST FOR
MILDLY MENTALLY RETARDED PERSONS

Population served: boys and girls, aged 8-18.

What Is Measured	Test Items
Arm and shoulder girdle strength	Flexed arm hang
Abdominal and hip flexor muscles	Sit-ups
Speed and agility	Shuttle run
Explosive muscular power	Standing long jump
Speed	50-yard dash
Skill and coordination	Softball throw for distance
Cardiovascular efficiency	300-yard run-walk

Source: The publication, *Special Fitness Test Manual for Mildly Mentally Retarded Persons*, which includes all the norms and details of tests, is available from American Alliance Publications, P.O. Box 704, Waldorf, Maryland 20601. Write for purchase information or order by phone: (703) 476-3481.

STANDARDIZED TESTS FOR
THE REGULAR POPULATION

The following physical fitness tests are designed for the regular population. Both of these tests may be adapted to serve selected disabled participants. Each instrument will indicate what is assessed and/or the test items.

AAHPER YOUTH FITNESS TEST

Population served: boys and girls, grades 5-12.

What Is Judged	Test Items
Arm and shoulder girdle strength	Pull-ups (boys) Flexed arm hang (girls)
Efficiency of abdominal and hip flexor muscles	Sit-ups (flexed legs)
Speed and change of direction	Shuttle run
Explosive muscular power of leg extensors	Standing broad jump
Speed	50-yard dash
Cardiovascular efficiency	600-yard run-walk 1-mile or 9-minute run, (ages 10-12) 1 1/2-mile or 12-minute run, (ages 13 and up)

Source: The publication, *AAHPER Youth Fitness Manual*, which includes all the norms and details of tests, is available from American Alliance Publications, P.O. Box 704, Waldorf, Maryland 20601. Write for purchase information or order by phone: (703) 476-3481.

HEALTH RELATED PHYSICAL FITNESS TEST

Population served: Youngsters, aged 5-18.

Components	Test Items
Cardiorespiratory function	Distance runs: 1-mile or 9-minute run 1 1/2-mile run or

Components	Test Items
	12-minute runs are optional for students 13 years or older
Sum of skinfold fat	Sum of the skinfolds of the triceps and subscapular
Abdominal muscular strength and endurance	Modified sit-ups
Flexibility (low back and posterior thighs)	Sit-and-Reach

Source: The publication, *AAHPERD Health Realted Physical Fitness Test Manual*, which includes all the norms and details of tests, is available from American Alliance Publications, P.O. Box 704, Waldorf, Maryland 20601. Write for purchase information or order by phone: (703) 476-3481.

USE OF COMPUTATION IN ASSESSMENT

The computer has the ability to make any job that requires large amounts of calculations or information processing easier. While this capability was originally available only to those with access to large, expensive computers, the microcomputer has moved this capability from the closed and often mysterious interior of the computer center into the hands of the user.

In the area of physical fitness test data, the computer can be of valuable use. Sports statistics, individual achievements, and other quantitative measures can be entered and compiled quickly and accurately by using the computer. Outcomes and projections can be made on relational input factors that allow for program planning and building into the future. Reports and other correspondence can be produced through a wide variety of word processing and text programs. Basically, anything that is presently being done by hand can most likely be done faster and more efficiently on a computer.

It is the purpose of this section to highlight some of the more useful types of computer applications for analysis and to provide some guidance as to what is necessary for successful utilization of computers in physical fitness work.

The Microcomputer

The microcomputer is a silicon chip capable of recording and storing strings of electronic impulses which act as the processing unit that directs all mathematical and instructional operations. This chip is also sometimes called a Central Processing Unit (CPU). The system of equipment commonly referred to as a microcomputer consists of one or more input devices (disk drive, cassette player, or keyboard, etc.), the CPU, one or more output devices (printer, video screen, etc.), and memory (the place where information is stored).

Memory is defined as either internal or external. The size of memory is measured in bits and bytes. One bit is equal to a positive or negative electronic charge. One byte is generally equivalent to eight bits and defines characters such as the number "1" or the literal "a" or "$." The letter "K" is used to define approximately 1000 bytes of memory (1024 to be exact). Thus 16k memory is approximately 16,000 characters of information. External memory is usually stored on magnetic tape or diskettes and measured in the same manner.

Internal memory comes in Read Only Memory (ROM) and Random Access Memory (RAM). ROM is reserved for the operating system and generally cannot be written over by the user. RAM is memory space that is available to, and controlled by, the user. Some microcomputers do not have a true ROM area and use part of RAM for the operating system. This is important if one is using a program which requires 44k of memory to run and the microcomputer available provides 48k of internal memory of which 8k is used for the operating system. Quick mathematics show that the operator is 4k of memory short to run both the operating system and the program.

Using the Computer

One can use the computer for almost anything that can be done with a pen, pencil, calculator or other conventional device for recording and manipulating information. The computer can be used for word processing; for information storage and retrieval, through readily available data base management programs that allow the creation and storage of information as needed; for data processing, by such programs as electronic spreadsheets and report writers that allow for retrieval and manipulation of data into a format that is designed and defined; the statistical analysis packages that are available to manipulate the data into analytical reports.

Through the use of these packages, which for the most part are available commercially through computer stores and software houses, such statistics as those provided by the AAHPER's "Motor Fitness Testing Manual for the Moderately Mentally Retarded" could be input into a microcomputer, data and statistical analysis procedures completed, and outcomes printed in a format most appropriate to one's needs.

Most computer sales people and many computer enthusiasts will try to tell the buyers that they just turn the computer on and within an hour they will be running programs as though it was something they had done all their lives. This will be especially true when purchasing commercially prepared programs.

It is true that the buyers will learn the basics of operating computers in a very short time. However, making effective use of the computers will take a little more effort. As with learning to type, the basics are simple. It's the speed and efficiency of using the typewriter that takes time and effort. However, when one has invested the necessary effort up front, the outcome will more than pay for the initial input.

And if an individual really doesn't have the time or desire to learn the ins and outs of using the microcomputer as an aid, he/she may want to enlist the help of someone who is adept at the use of computers. Investing in some programming from such a source and having it done by an expert may retrieve the information needed.

Getting Started

The instructor must first prioritize what he/she wants to use a computer for and estimate how much time is needed for each item. For example, for statistical analysis mainly, one needs equipment and software that will allow the easy input of necessary data and the easy retrieval of the analytical tables. Word processing would require a good word processing software program that has all the features needed, i.e., footnoting, superscript/subscript, spelling dictionary, etc., and a keyboard that is similar to a typewriter so as to allow for easy transition. Also of interest is whether or not the keyboard takes advantage of all the functions available in the software and vice versa.

Selecting the Right Equipment

If instructors want to get into microcomputers and need to look for equipment and programs, they should not go wrong if they follow these guidelines:

- First, the instructors need to decide what they want to do with a microcomputer.
- After they have decided, they should talk to users of computers, read some of the many magazines and books on the market, and visit some computer stores. (A good source of information might be a school computer science instructor.)
- Before they examine microcomputers, they should LOOK FOR THE SOFTWARE FIRST. No matter what microcomputer they like, it will do them no good if they are unable to find software to do what they want to do.
- After they have determined what they want to do, they should go to a computer store that has the software they want to see a demonstration of its operation on the microcomputer.
- When they find what they feel is a good software package, they should either buy or borrow the manual that goes with it. They should read it over thoroughly to see if they can understand it. If not, they should not purchase the software. It will do no good if they cannot use it.
- If they are unsure whether or not they are ready for using a computer, they should seek more advice on the matter.

Computers are one of the greatest tools available to humanity. Through them, fitness instructors can produce so much more in shorter periods of time. Computers can make lives easier and get rid of many of the humdrum, day-to-day tasks that tend to make work drudgery.

Instructors should be aware, however, that microcomputers can be frustrating, time-consuming, and useless if these persons are not ready and willing to invest some time into the care and nurturing of them.

Computing is for everyone; but not everyone is for computing.

That is something only each individual can decide. Investigating this resource carefully should precede the decision on the use of computers.

PRINCIPLES FOR ESTABLISHING INDIVIDUALIZED EXERCISE PRESCRIPTIONS FOR THE HANDICAPPED

Because of the many variables involved in prescribing exercise, an individualized approach to exercise prescription is imperative. Moreover, the needs and goals of each handicapped person who would like to start a fitness program must be considered.

The following guidelines must precede the discussion of principles for establishing individual exercise prescriptions:

* Complete medical records must be obtained in order to assess the individual's current health status. In addition, the type of medication taken, if any, must be known.
* Information concerning the person's present physical fitness level and exercise habits needs to be known. If not, such information must be established.
* Before he/she becomes involved in an exercise program, the individual's needs, interests, and objectives need to be analyzed.
* The person's short-term and long-term goals need to be established with objective criteria to see if these goals are realistic, i.e., objective, criteria for establishing progress.
* The instructor must provide sound advice regarding the proper clothing and equipment to be used in a fitness program.

If the instructor understands and practices the following principles, people with disabilities can improve their physical fitness capacity:

Type of Activity

Activities that produce good cardiovascular fitness are vigorous, continuous, and rhythmic; and they utilize the total body, for example running, walking, swimming, skiing. Heart rate response is the key to these types of activities. On the other hand, if muscular endurance, strength, and flexibility are desired, weight training and timed calisthenics are the types of activities that should be performed.

Intensity

The degree of difficulty is the key for cardiovascular and muscular strength and endurance improvement. With respect to cardiovascular fitness, target heart rate is related to energy cost; and it serves as an excellent tool for measurement.

The proper intensity may be calculated in two ways. First, the formula 220 minus the person's age; second; the Karvonen formula, which is 60-80 percent of the difference between the resting and maximal heart rates. However, researchers now claim that 75-85 percent of the difference between the resting and maximal heart rates is safe and gives both training effect and a method for monitoring activity levels. A quick pulse rate will indicate exercise rate if the pace has been continuous.

To determine pulse rate, one places two or three fingers of the opposite hand lightly on the radial artery located at the wrist behind the thumb, palm side, counts the pulsations for fifteen seconds, and multiples by four to find the number of beats per minute. A stop watch or wristwatch with a second hand is needed.

Duration

Duration is interrelated with intensity. In order to produce the required cardiovascular results, a specified amount of time is needed. At least 20-30 minutes of continuous physical activity are required to achieve cardiovascular benefits. If the duration of the exercise does not meet the time requirement, overloading is not sufficient to produce changes. Most handicapped beginners should start at a much lower level of duration than the above. Moreover, they must learn to adapt and progress slowly, as too much duration can cause over stress and possible injury.

Frequency

How often should handicapped people exercise? Initially, a good physical fitness program will require that the individual work out three or four times per week. Keep in mind that fitness cannot be stored; it must be renewed continuously.

Each exercise session requires the proper intensity and duration. Most people, if they adhere to the principle of frequency, will discover that improvements can be realized in between ten to twelve weeks. However, some handicapped individuals may wish to work out five to six times per week to get better and faster results.

Related Terminology

When discussing exercise prescriptions, instructors must familiarize themselves with these terms which are used frequently.

Overload

In order for one's body to improve, one must perform more work than he/she is normally accustomed to. The more conditioned people become, the harder it is for them to reach their target heart rates. Therefore, "overloading" is necessary in all fitness and physical conditioning programs. Gradually increasing the workload over a period of time will result in improved cardiovascular endurance or muscular strength and endurance predicated on the kind of fitness program undertaken.

Overloading can be accomplished in two ways: by increasing the **total work**, i.e., run further or play longer, and/or by increasing the **work rate**, i.e., run faster. With highly unconditioned individuals, overloading should be prescribed in small increments.

Progression

If one's body is to show improvement, one must be exposed to more and more intense levels of exercise. This advancement can be accomplished by the use of both overload and progression, as they are similar in nature. If a handicapped person stays at one particular fitness level, physiological adaptation takes place. This level is fine for fitness maintenance, but not for advancement for beginners or improved performance for athletes.

Use or Disuse

Simply stated, **use** promotes function while **disuse** promotes deterioration. The handicapped population often illustrate the concept of disuse. Viewing this population as a whole, one sees that, in general, they are too sedentary and should become more physically active.

Inactivity leads to poor muscle tone and strength and to decalcification of bones. X-rays of bones clearly demonstrate this decalcification in persons who are non-weight bearing. A similar x-ray finding is evident in those individuals who have a cast applied for a fractured leg, for example, and are immobile over a period of time. Therefore, weight-bearing should be reestablished as soon as possible and active exercise begun as soon as clinically indicated.

Specificity

The body responds differently to different activities imposed upon it. Thus, fitness improvements are specific to special training regimens.

A sound training program can use specificity for each component:

- Muscular strength and endurance results from weight training.
- Flexibility is derived from stretching and relaxation exercises.
- Cardiovascular endurance comes from aerobic activities.
- Body composition is the product of nutritional understanding and proper eating.

Specificity can be better accomplished from regular routines and not from random exercising.

Individual Differences

People with impairments, like other individuals, cannot be stereotyped because human beings respond differently to exercise. This fact is especially true when one is conducting an exercise program or choosing an exercise partner. Different factors such as risk factors and handicapping conditions will have a direct bearing on each individual. Examples:

- Obesity: (a major concern in exercise programs) Obese individuals usually need to lose weight first, then perhaps participate in a walk/jog program.

- Lower Back Rehabilitation: Individuals need slow progression exercises specifically designed to deal with the problem.
- Cardiac Rehabilitation: Individuals need certain specific kinds of exercises.
- Orthopedic Rehabilitation: Individuals usually need cycling and swimming.
- Injuries: Individuals need modification of program in addition to rehabilitation.

People exercise under all types of environmental conditions: extreme heat, cold, on and under water, and at various altitudes. Exercise physiologists have investigated all of these various conditions. As a result, an extensive body of knowledge is now available to people exercising under these varied conditions.

EXERCISE PRESCRIPTIONS

After all the fitness tests have been completed and the results have been analyzed, the instructor may write the exercise prescription. Care should be taken when developing prescriptions for individuals with handicapping conditions. Thus, the individualized approach must be used. The instructor is responsible for selecting the proper mode of activity since each individual will differ as to medical history, results of the physical examination, risk factors, as well as the present physical fitness status and exercise habits. Four sample exercise prescriptions may be found in Appendix A.

FITNESS COUNSELING

In addition to his/her other responsibilities, the fitness instructor should become involved with counseling handicapped individuals. Thus the holistic approach is pursued and the person's participation in physical fitness programs is better served. It would be helpful if the prospective counselor had some basic knowledge in guidance and counseling. However, when knowledge in these areas is lacking, the three most important attributes the instructor should possess are a comprehensive understanding of handicapping conditions, a realization of the individual's worth, and a strong desire and determination to help.

A counselor's function is to collect, organize, and analyze information about individuals through records, tests, and interviews in order to appraise their interests, aptitudes, abilities, personalities, and characteristics. Then he/she may better serve these individuals so that they enjoy exercising and make it a part of their lifestyle. Although the functions of the fitness counselor appear extensive, the keys to success are planning and organization.

Before attempting to counsel participants, instructors should first examine themselves through a series of questions:

- How do I perceive disabled persons?
- Do I understand handicapping conditions?
- Do I look upon all handicapped persons as having worth to themselves, their families, and to their communities?
- Do I have the proper attitude and personality necessary to counsel the disabled?
- Am I willing to devote my time and energy to helping handicapped people?
- Will I respect individuals for what they really are?
- Will I try to persuade handicapped persons to improve their physical and motor fitness levels?
- Will I allow disabled individuals to tell me about their own values and experiences?
- Will I be able to provide them with sound fitness counseling and advice?

It is of utmost importance that the prospective fitness counselor develop the following skills:

- Learn to perceive the handicapped participant as an equal.
- Learn to understand the participant's feelings and attitude toward physical activity.
- Learn to monitor the person's thoughts and words.
- Learn to respond in such a way as to make the disabled person feel comfortable and accept the message.
- Learn to understand the individual's message whether verbal or non-verbal. Look for hand, face, or other gestures.
- Learn to understand, through analysis, each person's physical

abilities and capacities.

- Learn to perceive individuals as independents capable of coping with their problems.
- Learn to counsel handicapped persons so that they understand their bodies and what their bodies are capable of doing.
- Learn to recognize negative self-concepts and poor body images.

Fitness counseling may be divided into six stages:

- Appraise: Collect data from various tests. Results from physical and motor fitness tests will be most helpful. Seek information from others if possible.
- Establish rapport: Get the participant to express his/her feelings of acceptance and understanding early in the first session.
- Reaffirm participant's firm belief in himself/herself.
- Listen intensely: Try to get persons to talk about their life experiences and their values.
- Respond appropriately: Think about what the participant said. Answer questions accurately and positively.
- Provide positive reinforcement: This task can be accomplished by repetition progress building of information related to physical fitness.
- Evaluate: Notes and records of each session should be kept, analyzed, and evaluated to determine if the individual's attitude and performance have changed.
- Do follow-up: Each counseling session should be followed up so that more data and information are collected which will assist the counselor in future sessions.

The handicapped, like their regular peers, are not immune from health-risk factors. One or any combination of these factors can contribute to sub-minimal physical fitness levels. Some fitness instructors may already be familiar with the eleven common health risk factors; however it seems prudent to repeat them here. The common health risk factors are overweight, underweight, poor nutrition, inadequate sleep and rest, respiratory problems, smoking, excessive use of drugs (not medications) and alcohol, stress, lack of physical activity, infectious diseases, and genetic factors.

In addition to the above risk factors, many disabled individuals have low physical fitness levels because they dislike physical activity.

They are afraid of failing, are embarrassed to perform, and do not like to perspire.

Fitness counseling, as it is associated with the disabled, may involve group counseling. The following eight group counseling techniques may prove helpful:

- The counselor should demonstrate an open concern with the problems that handicapped participants experience when starting a fitness program.
- Participants should have an opportunity to express openly their feelings about the physical activity.
- Factual information concerning the value of fitness programs and the long range effects such programs could have on their lives may be discussed in group sessions.
- There may be occasions of unpleasantness when participants are performing physical activities, especially in the early stages. These problems should be discussed.
- Assistance should be given in the setting of goals for the group in planning progressive steps to meet the goals of their fitness programs.
- Increased liking of physical activity should be reinforced by the counselor of the group.
- As participants familiarize themselves with the counselor and the group members and exhibit pride in improved performance, the counselor should point out the value of changes in their lifestyles.
- Once the participants have reached their established fitness goals, they should begin to re-evaluate themselves and establish new goals. Attainment of realistic goals is within reach if each member of the group is motivated to reach these goals.

Obviously, success in fitness counseling depends on both the participant and the counselor. The handicapped person must first learn to accept himself/herself as a human being capable of participating in a fitness program. Participants must make a commitment and be willing to change their lifestyles. They should be counseled to accept the fact that being physically fit will enable them to live a healthier, happier, and more productive life.

The major task confronting the counselor is to convince participants to start and continue a fitness program. Associated with the program is the exercise prescription designed specifically for each handicapped individual. Convincing people to exercise is not an easy task for the counselor, but perseverance by both parties will pay off. On the other hand, counselors should not expect every handicapped person to make exercise part of his/her lifestyle. There will be failures. There are those who will never be convinced that physical activity is beneficial. But the counselor should not get discouraged; there are many of the regular population who are not convinced either.

PROGRAM CONTRACTS

A program contract allows the intended participant to make an agreement with the instructor to complete a fitness program. But before the handicapped signs the contract, if possible, he/she must fully understand what it involves. The contract, although it appears to be confining and formal, is an excellent motivator.

Once they start, most disabled participants will have a tendency not to continue their fitness programs. The reasons usually given are that they are tired of exercising, are not feeling well, do not understand the benefits of exercise, are not mentally prepared to exercise, and that exercising takes too much time.

Four sample contracts of exercise programs may be found in Appendix B. They may be modified to meet the needs of participants with various types of disabling conditions.

Chapter VII

INSTRUCTING THE HANDICAPPED*

O F the several elements that comprise a quality fitness program for the handicapped, instruction should be first on the list. As instructors gain knowledge about disabling conditions, it is vital that they also learn how to teach this special population. Thus, this chapter will focus on instruction in the forms of methods, techniques, and suggestions.

The terms "method," "style," "strategy," "tactic," "mode," and "approach" are being used interchangeably to denote a procedure instructors employ to help participants learn. But, for the purpose of this section, the term "method" will be utilized. Method refers to a general, logical, organized, systematic instructional procedure. Basically, there are two general types of instructional methods — direct and indirect — with varying degrees in between. The direct method is traditional or instructor-centered, whereas the indirect method is problem-solving or participant-centered. In many cases, it is advisable to use a combination of both.

The term "technique," as used here, means a specific and comprehensive instructional procedure. Since they are the points of contact with the participant, these techniques must be taught in small units. They differ from method; they are more precise, more sensory, and more receptive to participant feedback. Because of this immediate feedback, individualized adjustments to learning problems receive on-the-spot attention. There are numerous techniques available to

---

*Adapted from Arthur G. Miller and James V. Sullivan, *op. cit.*, pp. 153-171.

instructors which can be applied to any of the methods, whether direct or indirect. Extensive treatment of teaching techniques related to physical fitness as they apply to both the regular and the special population may be found in the bibliography.

METHODS

Five instructional methods are recognized by educators and fitness practitioners. The direct methods are verbal, visual, kinesthetic, and tactile. These are instructor-centered, dictatorial, and one-way; moreover, there is little or no participant feedback.

A fifth method is called movement-exploration and is classified as two-way; it allows for maximum participant feedback. In theory, these five instructional methods are separate; however, in practice, they are used in combinations. It is the fitness instructor's resourcefulness and teaching ability that can help to create a positive learning climate.

Verbal

The most direct method of teaching is verbal, wherein the instructor primarily utilizes spoken words to describe what is to be learned, how it is to be performed, and what response is expected from the performance. The major merits of this method are that it permits a quick "laying-out" of the instruction, and it provides identification of each element of the total activity, including descriptions of internal and external cues. In presenting the verbal method, instructors should keep in mind certain cautions. First, if the participant is mentally retarded, instructors should use simple language, speak slowly and directly, and be as unambiguous as possible. Moreover, the instructors' vocabularies must be free of abstractions, and sentence structure must be uninvolved. Instruction then must be in concrete terms, given clearly and distinctly, and sprinkled with humor and imagination in order to hold the attention of those participants with short attention spans.

Visual

The visual method of teaching utilizes demonstration so that the participant can see what the "model" to be learned looks like. The model is presented in perfect form so that it can be copied by the participant and needs no translation into words. For most retarded participants who have difficulty in developing visual images from words, using the visual method is imperative. A disadvantage of this method, however, is that the kinesthetic part of the exercise or activity cannot be communicated back to the instructors.

There are several ways, in addition to demonstration, for participants to visualize an exercise or activity. Various kinds of instructional media are available — films, filmstrips, loopfilms, slides, photo enlargements, posters, and diagrams. The combination of both film and videotape is now being widely used for teaching exercises and fitness activities to the handicapped.

After a film of an exercise or fitness activity has been seen, participants imitate it while a video camera records their performance. Afterwards, participants see themselves on a videotape projection and draw comparisons between perfect performance and their own. For some, the original film and the videotape are strong motivators; for others, the gap between the ideal and the real is so great that motivation lessens.

Visual aids attract the handicapped, especially when the performance that they have seen involves other disabled individuals. After they realize that the models themselves have similar handicapping conditions, they may put forth more effort than usual during the fitness sessions.

Instructors should encourage their participants to bring clippings from newspapers and magazines that depict an exercise or fitness activity which they would like to "copy." To reinforce learning, instructors can display these pictorial materials on a bulletin board that can be seen frequently. For example, pictures that show good running form can be placed in sequence on a bulletin board.

Participants can pick up terminology related to physical fitness from other printed material, such as books, periodicals, pamphlets, and newspaper clippings. But instructors should keep in mind that instructional media are not substitutes for the relationship between themselves and their participants.

Kinesthetic

In contrast to the verbal and visual methods is the kinesthetic method, one that is intended to provide sensory data that the participant could not acquire in any other way about the exercise or activity to be learned. Kinesthesia may be defined as a sense mediated by end organs located in muscles, tendons, and joints which stimulates bodily movements and tensions. Words, pictorial materials, and demonstrations cannot communicate the sensory data; it must be experienced by the participant through movement.

Two examples may help instructors understand this kinesthetic method better. In a class that consists of four multihandicapped youngsters with both cerebral palsy and mental retardation, the instructor wishes to teach the proper body mechanics for walking. Although these youngsters were given time to look at pictures of walking and to listen to the description of the bodily movements associated with activity, their responses were poor. The instructor has the youngsters stand on a line and manually assists each one through the proper sequence of walking. After all have had an opportunity to walk, the instructor allows them to walk unassisted and asks them if they can "feel" the movements of each step. This procedure is done several times both assisted and unassisted. Each time the youngsters walk unassisted, the instructor evaluates and again asks whether they can recognize the correct "feeling" of each step.

An analysis of teaching trainable mentally retarded individuals how to perform sit-ups may better illustrate this kinesthetic method. In a fitness class consisting of six participants, three are positioned lying on their backs on mats, fingers lightly grasping the head, covering the ears. Knees are bent, feet flat on the mat and slightly apart. Three participants hold down both ankles of the three who are performing the sit-ups. The back is curled up and the trunk is raised until the trunk is vertical to the floor and both elbows touch the thighs. As this action is taking place, the instructor asks whether participants can feel the tension or "pull" on stomach muscles and the pressure on the hip joints. As the three curl up, the instructor can point out that pressure on the stomach is to be expected. Similary, as the individuals return to their starting positions, they will again feel tension on the abdominal muscles as well as on the tendons and hip joints. After a few sit-ups have been performed, the learners gradually come to acquire the correct "feel" of the entire sit-up sequence. After the three have performed the sit-up sequence, the three ankle holders go through the same learning routine.

Authorities have cited two drawbacks to the kinesthetic method. First, many handicapped participants lack "body awareness." Taking movement for granted, they have difficulty identifying muscular tension. Instructors should repeatedly point out **which** movements produce **which** effects.

A second drawback relates to fitness instructors. The correctness of an exercise or activity will suffer unless the instructor has sufficient time to keep the participant's attention on performing satisfactorily. The kinesthetic method requires full attention of both the learner and the instructor. Unless both give their deep concentration to the exercise or activity, the participant will find performing independently difficult. In other words, some understanding of how muscles contract and extend in movement is helpful in the performance of an exercise or fitness activity. Thus the participant needs to become familiar with muscular actions proper to the correct movements or "models."

Tactile

The tactile method involves the ability to recognize and interpret one's environment without vision — by touching, rubbing, pressing, or manipulating. Usually this process is carried out by using the fingers and encompasses kinesthetic (internal) and tactile (external) sensations which are transmitted to the brain. The ability to recognize objects by touch is vital not only to the handicapped but also to the non-handicapped as well.

The tactile method is used successfully with the blind and the retarded. Instructors working with the blind rely heavily on this method. Since the retarded have problems in conceptualizing, they are receptive to using the tactile approach. Fitness teachers working with the blind are encouraged to use both the tactile and verbal methods; but with the retarded, all methods warrant experimentation.

Although fitness exercise with a light dumbbell may start out as passive, it may become active. Instructed merely to hold the dumbbell, a blind youngster may be asked to feel, rub, and manipulate it and eventually perform an arm curl. The passive tactile method, when combined with the active, expands the possibility of ennumberable exercises and fitness activities.

Movement Exploration

A fifth method, movement exploration, is the only indirect method used by fitness instructors. Primarily used in settings that allow for freedom of movement, it is participant-centered and not instructor-centered. According to their capacities, handicapped individuals are given the freedom and responsibility to set their own goals, to make a selection of exercises and activities, to perform these exercises and activities in their own way, to set their own pace, to select assistance from any source, and when possible, to self-evaluate. Instructor-initiated visual demonstrations or models are temporarily discontinued, as are commands and instructions usually associated with the verbal method. Problem-solving questions and suggestions are utilized to initiate movement exploration and to stimulate the exercise or activity upon which participants can build. The participants, however, must take the initiative of comparing their own performances with those of their peers, when possible.

Although instructors will develop their own style of presentation of problem-solving situations, the following phrases and words have proven successful: "Who can _____?" "How can _____?" "What other ways _____?" "With whom can you _____?" The answers to these questions or problems which have been raised are in the form of movements rather than words. Each participant moves in his or her own way, with the interpretation or answer to the challenge probably being different for each person. With no "right" or "wrong" response being expected, individuals are free to express themselves as they interpret the problem and are able to progress at their own rate.

A sample of a movement exploration lesson follows that may help instructors better to understand this method: A special group of seven- to ten-year olds might be asked a question which encourages physical activity: "How can you make yourself bigger?" The responses range from simple gestures to moving arms and legs in all directions. One youngster may expand his stomach, while another youngster may attempt to form a human "X." Someone else runs around in a circle. The instructor continues by saying, "Can you make yourselves smaller and smaller?" Kneeling down, curling in a ball, hiding arms and legs and head are the responses. Again, the instructor, "Show me the ways that you get from here to the corners of the gym." Some youngsters crawl or creep; others walk, run, jump, or skip; others even go backward or sideward. After this, the instructor may continue by saying, "Now show me a different way from the one you used before to get from here to the corners of the gym" — a suggestion that challenges youngsters as well as makes them think. In short, fitness instructors will soon realize that movement exploration expands the participants' potential for exercise and physical activity and creates amusement, instills self-confidence, and makes them aware of a variety of bodily movements within their capabilities.

Combining Methods

The examples that follow are intended to illustrate two or more of the five methods combined to teach one exercise or activity. Few, if any, activities would encompass use of all five methods of instruction for a given exercise or activity.

A typical lesson that combines verbal, visual, and movement-exploration methods may involve having participants choose an object from a group of supplies placed at the center of the gymnasium floor (hula hoop, tire, jump rope, dowel, and medicine ball). The instructor says, "What have you chosen? . . . Describe it for me . . . Now, show me how to use it . . . What else can you do with it?" Most individuals will respond with some type of physical expression. Those who do not, may seek aid from a peer or hints and clues from the instructor.

Acting out the movements of a jogger, weight-trainer, or aerobic dancer stimulates movement exploration in bodily expression. The instructor begins by saying, "Be a jogger . . . First do several stretching exercises . . . Now take a starting position, one foot ahead of the other . . . On the command 'ready, set, go' start to jog . . . Move both your legs and your arms as you jog . . . Now you should be in a correct jogging form!" If a participant hesitates, the instructor resorts to verbal instructions that are reinforced, if necessary, by visual aids. A sequence of sketches or pictures of handicapped individuals jogging may prove helpful; and in some instances, music spurs creativity.

When verbal and visual instruction are purposely withdrawn, however, the results may be mixed: Some persons, if left to their own initiative, show style and confidence, while others are inactive. It should be remembered that to impose the exploratory method on participants with mental or physical disabilities may simply be unrealistic. For individuals to be instructed on how to perform the movements of a jogger, no single method should be utilized.

In an adapted physical fitness class, three have mild cerebral palsy, one has a deformed arm, one's arm has been amputated, one wears braces, and two are partially deaf. In a game of circle dodgeball, everyone should be given a chance to see just what goes on: Where the teams stand, how the ball is put into play, and why the players move as they do. A combination of teaching methods, the instructor soon learns, is vital.

After the count-off, each team member is allowed to show how he or she dodges the ball while staying inside the circle. The three participants with cerebral palsy and the one wearing braces may have difficulty moving, but they move as fast as they can. The two partially deaf, who frequently lose their balance during the game, are shown how to widen their stances and crouch low for stability. The game of circle dodgeball has thus given the instructor an opportunity to utilize the verbal, visual, and movement-exploratory methods as well as the kinesthetic method.

TECHNIQUES

Given all that has been previously said about methods, instructors who are eager to learn may ask, "Where should I start?" or "At what point do I switch from methods to techniques?" The answers to these two questions should be delayed until the instructor has had an opportunity to review the nature and degree of the handicapping conditions and the ability, both actual and potential, of the participants.

For example, for most disabled participants, learning how to perform progressive resistance exercises requires a general **method** of instruction. For our purpose here, the stages of this introductory method on how to perform one exercise, arm (biceps) curls on a weight-training machine are roughly these:

- "Stand near (or bring the wheelchair close) facing the machine."

- "Grip the handle tightly with both hands."
- "Adjust the grip, if necessary."
- "To begin, keep both arms extended."
- "Flex the arms."
- "Extend the arms."
- "Breathe freely."
- "Good! Try again."

The difference between the above **method** of, and **techniques** for, instructing the same exercise of fitness activity is a matter of specificity and precision. An abundance of details is available to participants who are ready for the complexities of techniques.

Starting Position

Participant stands up straight (or sits in a wheelchair) about one foot away from the arm curl station on the weight-training machine, facing it with feet apart equal to shoulder width. Toes are pointed directly ahead at the station and are parallel. In the "ready" position, the handle is held in front of the body at thigh level by fully extending the arms. Eyes are focused straight ahead as the participant awaits the command "lift."

Grip

Both hands, palms upward, grip the handle with the fingers comfortably spread apart. The hands are spaced the width of the shoulders. If too far apart, bring both hands in one inch toward the center of the handle.

Lift

In "ready" position, the participant has weight equally distributed on both feet. Arms are fully flexed, elbows close to, but not touching, the sides. The handle is brought to the chest and held in that position for three seconds. Weights are returned slowly, the arms are fully extended, and the handle is touching the thighs. The breath must not be held; breathing should be rhythmical.

Techniques, in contrast to methods, reflect in detail the ultimate complexity of an exercise or a fitness activity from which briefer, more general, methods are derived. Instructors sometimes ask, "What difference does it make whether I use methods or techniques? Is there some practical advantage that one approach has over the other?" While it is true that the finer points of an exercise or fitness activity may be lost to some participants, these points should not be lost to the instructor. After all, many disabled individuals may benefit from merely seeing or hearing technical details about an exercise or a fitness activity.

At this point in the discussion, it may be advisable to explain the relationship of technique to method, a part-to-whole relationship. Once the disabled person has performed a part of a total response (an exercise or fitness activity), this performance tends to improve motivation. Acquiring a second, and then a third, sub-response may motivate the participant into an accumulation of sub-responses that open up the possibility of learning the total exercise or activity in correct sequence. Thus he/she may perform this exercise (activity) with better timing and coordination.

It is recommended that participants should first be taught exercises and fitness activities by utilizing methods; then, by techniques. To withhold techniques altogether would deny disabled participants a right to know, to aspire, and to find success as they progress in individualized fitness activities and programs.

The eager instructor may ask the question, "How many and what kinds of techniques should be offered in a fitness program?" The answer may seem obvious, but every stage of the participant's developmental pattern should benefit from the appropriate exercise or activity. Furthermore, most personnel working with the handicapped believe in meeting the individual's need "where they are." Conversely, there are those who emphasize fixed standards regardless of the constant change in performance levels; its proponents attempt to seek mastery of exercises and activities through adherence to proper techniques. The conscientious instructor is convinced that training and practice can provide the participant with deep satisfaction.

Instructors who are eager to move into techniques may ask:

- "If I teach all the techniques of an exercise or fitness activity, how much time should I devote to each type?"
- "What degree of motor learning can I expect from each participant?"

- "Is it better to teach techniques to an individual or to a group?"

All three questions are unanswerable unless the instructor has developed a philosophy and a firm knowledge of each participant's disabling condition. These can be acquired only by working steadily and observing closely; without question, the best strategy is through methods, while techniques are delayed until the foundation is laid relative to the needs, interests, and goals of each participant.

Breaking down any motor task into its separate components and identifying each in relation to the whole task is known as **task analysis.** Such an analysis is the most effective way to determine whether or not a participant has progressed in the sequence thoroughly enough to go on to more complex tasks. For a handicapped participant, the mere act of lifting only the handle of a weight-training machine or only a bar over the head requires some strength and control. Similarly, some handicapped persons cannot perform the above motor task unless the instructor has guided them **through** the movements. In both instances, the instructor analyzes and teaches such basic fundamentals as body position, hand grip, balance, and total body control.

In learning how to perform weight-training exercises, a young handicapped individual can receive various degrees of help by direct manual guidance and by the use of prosthetic devices. The appropriateness of the individual techniques depends on an accurate task analysis.

If a twelve-year-old Down's syndrome youngster tries without success to perform a sitting windmill, which is a flexibility or stretching exercise, he/she obviously needs someone who has analyzed this exercise for what it is — a series of sub-tasks:

- Sit on the mat and spread your legs out as far as you can.
- Put your hands out to your sides and keep your back straight.
- Touch your right hand to your left foot (knee-shin).
- Return to your starting position.
- Touch your left hand to your right foot (knee-shin). Return to your starting position.
- Keep your arms and legs straight at all times.
- Repeat these movements to opposite sides.

When the youngster has learned the above components identified in the task analysis, his/her progress in performing a sitting windmill will improve. Furthermore, if the exercise was given a predetermined time table to complete a fixed number of repetitions, after a period of work-outs, the youngster would improve in muscular strength and endurance.

SUGGESTIONS FOR INSTRUCTION APPLICABLE TO SPECIFIC HANDICAPS

Fitness instructors may find the following information helpful when teaching those with specific handicapping conditions.

Visual Handicaps

Blind participants will explore unfamiliar objects and react in one or two ways: Either they will associate the tactile sensation with a previous experience and quickly identify the object, or they will go through a complex mental process not entirely understood by psychologists. Usually they reduce the alternatives until an identification is made. In the event they do not, blind individuals may become frustrated and defeated. Thus it is important that pieces of equipment or items of supplies that are to be used by blind participants be clearly described as to color, texture, size, and shape. It is also important to synchronize the examination of an object by the participant with the full description of it by the instructor.

Whenever possible, the participant should be helped to "feel" and follow the movements of a sighted participant or the instructor. This task is accomplished by placing one or both hands on the sighted person's arms, waist, legs, or feet.

All instructions should be given slowly so that all participants can understand the exercise or fitness activity as well as memorize its location indoors, outdoors, or in the pool.

Whenever possible, it is a good idea to have the participants join a sighted companion in a physical fitness activity to add both incentive and the acquisition of skill and knowledge.

The manner in which instructors speak to blind participants is extremely important. Their attitude and tone of voice often communicate as much as, if not more than, the words spoken. A reassuring tone may result in a positive response, whereas dull instruction may be disregarded.

The word "see" is often used when speaking to blind people. They know it means "understand."

Participants should always be kept informed of the location of both their peers and the instructor.

Auditory communication may be encouraged by helping participants identify themselves by name and to use the names of their companions. When sighted participants speak, their peers will soon recognize their voices.

The two best approaches to use with the blind are verbal instructions and manual assistance. Both should be given equal time.

Because of the auditory acuity of the blind, various sounds are helpful, particularly if they are produced near the object which is to be identified and learned. For example, metal keys or metal objects can be secured under the center section of a trampoline bed to help a participant jog in place near the center of the bed. These jogging movements, performed over a period of time, will improve the individual's cardiovascular endurance.

Various types of audible balls with sound mechanisms should be used for fitness activities and games. These balls are now available and may be purchased from American Foundation for the Blind, 15 West 16th Street, New York, New York, 10011, or from some sporting goods stores.

Music, as an accompaniment to various tempos and rhythms, should be used when teaching aerobic dance movements and patterns. However, the music must not be so loud as to interfere with instruction.

Blind participants should never be left "stranded." If they need to be left alone for a short while, explain to them exactly where they are. A rule of thumb to follow is to place them in contact with a wall, fence, or a piece of equipment. Moreover, they should be given their canes in the event they need to leave the immediate area.

In a pool, it is essential that all types of floatation aids and ropes be used for both safety and instruction.

Auditory Handicaps

If fitness instructors choose to work with the deaf, they should learn both sign language and lip reading. It is also beneficial that they learn how to interpret facial expressions and eye and body movements. Courses in communications with the deaf and hard of hearing are offered in colleges and universities.

Instructors should learn to pronounce their words clearly and speak slowly so that their lips may be read. The best location for speaking is in front of the fitness class so all can see. The activity area should be free from distracting sounds.

Visual aids of all kinds should be utilized, such as chalkboards, diagrams, slides, films, loop films and videotapes.

It is best to offer new exercises or fitness activities from start to finish, the whole method, as the deaf rely heavily on visual acuity.

Deaf participants usually learn best when they are taught in small groups, where social interaction may be enhanced.

Schedule a variety of balancing (mostly dynamic) fitness activities such as walking along strips of masking tape placed on the floor, walking on a low balance beam, and bouncing on a mini or regular trampoline. These types of activities help to compensate for the poor equilibrium of the deaf and can help them gain cardiovascular endurance.

Neuromuscular and Orthopedic Handicaps

Competitive fitness activities should be avoided completely or kept at a minimum.

Do not offer exercises or activities that require time limits, as many of these participants are nervous and cannot cope with pressure. Just getting them to participate will be an accomplishment.

Offer wheelchair-bound participants an opportunity to exercise and to take part in activities within their capabilities. All movements performed to music may be interpreted as dance. Encourage them to bend and extend their bodies and body parts within their limitations.

Offer these participants all types of fitness programs, using adaptations, when necessary.

Cardiovascular Handicaps

The instructor must consider the principles of exercise — mode of activity, intensity, duration, and frequency — involved in each fitness activity and both its immediate and long-range effects when working with participants who have cardiovascular disabilities.

Avoid such rapid exercises as arms overhead, arms extended outward, arm circles, or jumping jacks as they may induce stress and overtax the heart.

Throwing or lifting heavy objects should be avoided. Do not offer runs or walks for speed or distance nor climbing under demanding conditions.

Avoid intensive competitive activities, participation in too vigorous activities, or prolonged activities.

Respiratory Handicaps

Progressive resistance exercises, when used properly, strengthen the respirtory muscles. Breathing exercises performed in various body positions should be offered frequently.

Over-competitive activities which may produce fatigue and emotional stress should be avoided.

Swimming should be encouraged as a means of utilizing all muscle groups and strengthening the entire respiratory system, thereby improving cardiorespiratory endurance.

Mental Handicaps

Use demonstrations or models and reduce verbal explanations. The retarded like to mimic; follow-the-leader exercises and activities should be used. If verbal instructions are used, they should be concrete, not abstract. Remember, these persons have short attention spans.

Motivating these participants to exercise and take part in fitness activities may be a major task.

When appropriate, provide music as a motivator.

Praise generally produces a better reaction than a reprimand; the recognition of a participant's success in an exercise or fitness activity is important.

Obstacle courses are of interest and within the capability of the retarded participant if the courses are properly set up and produce the desired fitness results.

Severely and profoundly retarded participants should be taught simple locomotion movements — crawling, creeping, walking, and, for some, running — but other fitness activities such as roller skating with the aid of a walker, pushing a moon-buggy in a relay race, and tricycling are excellent fitness activities.

Emotional Handicaps

Short attention spans are inevitable; when the doldrums set in, the instructor should be ready with alternatives.

Do not rush these participants, as they are withdrawn, shy, fearful, and/or hypersensitive. If possible, a good approach is to have them watch their peers in action and encourage them to imitate.

Younger autistic participants usually need manual guidance.

These participants should not be expected to stay in one position or be confined in a small area for any length of time.

Do not offer several strenuous exercises or fitness activities in succession.

Instructors should learn to recognize and anticipate gestures, facial expressions, and body movements as well as other participant reactions.

Upsets and seizures may be induced by sudden noises; these must be avoided.

It is best to offer exercises and fitness activities that all participants can perform; however, provisions should be made for alternatives.

Chapter VIII

KNOWING ABOUT FITNESS
PROGRAMS AND ADAPTATIONS

A S mentioned previously, participants wishing to enter a fitness program must have completed a medical examination and received clearance before the fitness assessment can be administered. Upon completion of this assessment, the exercise prescription is developed. After the preceding steps have been completed, instructors are now assured that their participants are ready to begin individualized fitness programs.

The first section of this chapter will provide fitness instructors with a general description of fitness programs for the regular population. Each program will be briefly described and placed under one or more physical or health-related fitness components, where appropriate. The titles of fitness books which contain methods and techniques of instruction for the regular population may be found in the bibliography.

The second section of this chapter will include factors involved in adapting instruction, guidelines for making adaptations, suggested adaptations as they relate to exercises, activities, or programs. Additionally, a brief description of three adapted fitness programs will be presented. Titles of fitness books which contain methods and techniques of instruction may be found in the bibliography.

Note: See Appendix C for a Suggested Listing Of Physical Fitness Activities Classified By Major Component Provided For The Instructor.

Fitness programs are usually designed to encompass all five of the physical or health-related components: cardiovascular endurance, muscular strength, muscular endurance, flexibility, and body fat composition. Moreover, the beginning instructor must be cognizant of the fact that each program should be structured to focus upon the development of one or more specific components and include others as part of the program. For example, walk/jog emphasizes the development of cardiovascular endurance; weight training and timed calisthenics emphasize the development of muscular strength and endurance, and static stretching exercises emphasize the development of flexibility. Yet walk/jog also increases muscular strength and endurance, and warm-up exercises for weight training and timed calisthenics also increase flexibility. Body fat composition, although a fitness component, is interrelated with all types of fitness programs. Individuals who exercise regularly and have sensible eating habits usually maintain satisfactory weight control.

CARDIOVASCULAR ENDURANCE

All the programs described below are aimed at developing cardiovascular endurance or aerobic capacity.

Aerobic Dance

Aerobic Dance is a choreographed exercise program which is concerned primarily with developing cardiovascular endurance, but it also increases muscular endurance and flexibility. Relaxation exercises are also included in an aerobic dance program. Sessions usually are organized to consist of warm-ups, aerobic conditioning, cool down, and relaxation exercises. Aerobic conditioning is accomplished through simple dances that range from slow, stretching warm-ups to strenuous, rhythmical routines. This workout pattern is followed by exercises performed on mats to improve muscle tone, muscle strength, and flexibility. Moreover, the development of proper body mechanics and maximum range of motion are integral parts of the program. Finally, various muscular relaxation exercises complete each session. All the above mentioned elements, combined with music and dance, offer participants much fun, challenge, and a feeling of well-being.

Aquatic Fitness

Aquatic Fitness is a complete cardiovascular program for those who prefer swimming for exercise. Non-swimmers may also enroll in these types of programs as there are a variety of non-swimming exercises which can be performed at the shallow end of a pool. Although any stroke or combination of strokes may be used, it is generally advisable to have the participants begin with the resting strokes, such as breaststroke, sidestroke, and elementary backstroke, until they become accustomed to the workout routine; then they may employ more vigorous strokes.

Each aquatic exercise class should contain three main components:

- A combination warm-up/water calisthenics routine performed in the shallow end of the pool,
- A peak exercise period to elevate heartrates to improve cardiorespiratory endurance (swimming, shallow water walking exercises, bobbing, kicking, and watergames), and
- A cool-down period of slow walking and swimming and final stretch-downs on the pool deck.

Interval Training

Interval Training is an aerobic type program whereby participants exercise continuously and strenuously for a period of time and rest for a period of time. Its major aim is to increase progressively the exercise work load and to decrease the time of rest periods.

Although interval training was first utilized in running, it can be used in other activities such as fast walking, swimming, or cycling. Some fitness experts believe that each exercise period should last for five minutes and each rest period one minute and that there should be a minimum of six exercise periods performed every other day.

Exercise work load may be increased by:

- Increasing the distance of the activity
- Increasing the speed of the activity
- Increasing the number of times the activity is performed.

Rest periods may be decreased by shortening the time of each period or by changing the intensity of the activity during the rest period. For example, participants may run more slowly, walk more slowly, swim more slowly, or cycle more slowly during the so-called rest periods.

Walk/Jog

Walk/Jog is an exercise program designed for people who have been sedentary or who otherwise are not in good physical condition. Most of these types of programs have been based on the "Y's Way to Fitness," a nationwide program of cardiovascular endurance training.

Each class session in a typical walk/jog program consists of the resting pulse rate, warm-ups, peak work-out, target pulse rate, cool down, relaxation exercises, and the post-exercise pulse rate. These programs are usually divided into ten-week sessions, and individuals start as beginners. Each class session should begin very slowly and progress a little during each of the following weeks. At the end of ten weeks, participants may elect to go into the intermediate program. After this program, they may wish to continue into the advanced program. Instructors should be advised, moreover, that with entry into each new level of the program, participants are developing cardiovascular endurance as well as improving muscular strength and endurance.

Outdoor Fitness

A parcourse fitness circuit is a program designed to provide participants with stretching exercises and strengthening and toning exercises. In conjunction with these exercises performed at the designated stations, walking and/or jogging complete the course. Some people use a parcourse for cycling or in the wintertime in some parts of the country, for skiing and snowshoeing.

A parcourse fitness program can accommodate all levels of participants, that is, beginners, intermediates, and advanced, or well conditioned athletes. A parcourse is unique because at each station a "par" system is available which recommends the number of exercises considered par according to the level of the participant.

At the start of the parcourse is a "heart check guide" which explains the idea of the pulse-rated exercise. At the first station, participants may find their "exercise heart rate range." As they continue through the course, they come upon "heart check" stations spaced throughout the circuit. These serve as reminders to check pulse rates.

The description of how to perform each exercise is posted at every station. Also at each station is an outline figure of an individual demonstrating the proper way the exercise should be performed. Once participants begin the use of a parcourse fitness circuit and stay with the program, they will discover it is very beneficial and enjoyable.

MUSCULAR STRENGTH AND ENDURANCE

The following are designed to develop muscular strength and endurance.

Weight Training

Weight training, or progressive resistance exercise, is a program utilizing assorted weights, either barbells and dumbbells, or weight-training machines for performing exercises. A sound weight-training program should follow a developmental pattern and should be programmed to meet the specific physical needs of the individual.

A basic weight-training program should include most of the major muscle and muscle groups, and there should be at least three work-outs a week. The participants should perform three sets (a stated number of repetitions) of exercises during the sessions and take a five-minute rest between each set. Each exercise should be performed eight to ten repetitions (going through the full exercise one time). The amount of weight used depends on the physical status of the participant. Beginners should always start with a light load and add weights as they progress. All exercises should be performed without straining.

Circuit Training

Circuit weight training, as described here, is designed to allow a large number of participants to perform a variety of exercises during the same weight-training session. A circuit is formulated which contains several different exercise stations. With this type of organization, the individual may perform alone or be part of a group or class. Circuit training, however, can be constructed with exercise stations, so that a variety of fitness activities may be performed with little or no equipment.

Circuit training may be used successfully with either men and women or boys and girls. Because this type of training is very adaptable, the exercise stations may cover a variety of situations and still allow for individual differences among a group or class. Furthermore, several people can exercise in a short period of time, yet each person performs according to his/her individual needs and ability.

The advantages of circuit training are as follows:

- Although the instructor diagnoses the person's deficiencies, the participant may, however, assist the instructor in choosing the exercises he/she is required to perform. Careful selection of exercises is important.
- Because of the adaptability of the exercise stations, individuals usually find most of them suitable. In some cases, improvisations may be necessary with some of the equipment.
- Since this type of training is based on the overload principle, each person's workload is set on an individual basis.
- Progression depends on the participant's ability to execute the exercises prescribed before taking on an additional load. Furthermore, each individual in the group or class is designated at a particular point on a continuum and, hopefully, progresses from that point.
- Each participant's working toward his/her personal goal should provide for a positive self-concept as well as act as a motivator to achieve the goal.
- Workloads, repetitions, and time frames are an integral part of this type of program and thus they tend to help the underdeveloped person toward a satisfactory physical fitness level.
- Because the exercise stations are highly organized, a whole group may complete the circuit in a short period of time. However, some individuals may need assistance at some stations.
- Usually, six to eighteen exercise stations comprise a complete circuit. However, any number of stations may be utilized to

meet the needs of the group or class.

- As each participant will be on an individualized exercise program, he/she should know what exercises to perform and should be required to execute them to the best of his/her ability.
- A circuit training program has potential in meeting the participant's physical and motor needs. It will be beneficial to him/her only if the program is implemented properly.

Timed Calisthenics

A Timed Calisthenics program can be designed to help participants develop muscular strength and endurance. At every class session, the participant performs the exercises repetitiously and increases the number of exercises performed within a predetermined time interval. For example, as a beginner who is in poor physical condition, a person may perform five sit-ups in one minute. At the third class, the same person may perform seven sit-ups in one minute and gradually increase the number until he/she is capable of performing a satisfactory number of sit-ups in a specified number of minutes.

When presenting timed calisthenics, the instructor should start with exercises for the neck and work down to the toes. In addition, exercises should be given that include the total body and body parts. Timed calisthenic classes should meet at least three times a week, for a period of twelve weeks. Each class session should be at least forty minutes in length and consists of stretching, timed calisthenics (peak conditioning period), cool-down, and relaxation exercises.

FLEXIBILITY

Static stretching exercises may be utilized to develop flexibility. Each exercise should be sustained for five to seven seconds. When these exercises are presented in a series, they comprise a program. In some instances, selected flexibility exercises sometimes referred to as warm-ups, precede any training or work-out session because it is at this time that the muscles and joints of the body need to be loosened and stretched. Many people lack overall flexibility because they do not use certain muscles and joints in their daily lives.

Flexibility exercise classes should meet three or four times a week, each class being at least thirty minutes in length. These classes should continue for at least ten weeks. Participants should be instructed to perform the various exercises slowly and **not bounce** in an attempt to stretch further (called ballistic stretching). Gaining a satisfactory level of overall flexibility takes time and patience. For some it may be advisable to use a combination of flexibility exercises and some type of cardiovascular endurance activity.

Obviously, muscular relaxation is not a physical or health-related fitness component. It is included in this section, however, because relaxation exercises are utilized in most fitness programs. The teaching of relaxation exercises should be an integral part of most fitness programs. Although utilized as only the culmination of these programs, relaxation exercises are very beneficial to participants since these techniques bring about a conscious release of muscle tension.

In response to the need to learn how to escape from the effects of stress and tension, relaxation exercises have played an important role. The stiffness of the muscles and joints of tense people is a direct result of stress. In late stages, stress and tension may cause the joints to become so tight that flexibility may not be regained.

When utilized as a part of fitness programs, relaxation exercises are presented at the end of each class and take up approximately five to seven minutes of class time. Generally, ten exercises are provided per class and are aimed at muscles of the neck, arms, fingers, shoulders, trunk, hips, legs, feet, and toes. There are many muscular relaxation exercises available.

Most of the instruction in relaxation is verbal, but there may be instances when each technique may need to be demonstrated. If indoor mats are provided, the lights should be turned off, the exercise area should be quiet, and the instructors should speak as softly as possible.

ADAPTATIONS

Adaptation, as used in this context, refers to changing or modifying either assessment, instruction, exercises, activities, programs, equipment, supplies, facilities, or any single one or combination of these. Obviously, the main reason that adaptations are made is to accommodate individuals with handicapping conditions. However, it is not intended here to discuss all of the types of adaptations that are listed above but to focus only on exercises, activities, and programs.

Sherrill, (1981) in her book reveals that "adapting instruction to the needs and interests of students is mostly a matter of common sense and creativity. A knowledge of biomechanical and fitness principles helps also."[1]

She also states: "Adapting involves manipulating the factors that affect the teaching/learning process. Some of the factors are:

- Teaching style
- Verbal instructions
- Demonstration
- Level of methodology
- Starting and stopping signals
- Time of day, season of year
- Duration
- Order of learning or trials
- Pupil-teacher ratios
- Size of group
- Nature of group
- Instructional setting
- Equipment
- Architectural barriers and distance of playing area from classrooms
- Level of difficulty/complexity
- Motivation"[2]

An adapted exercise or physical fitness activity is one that has been modified or adjusted to fit the functioning levels of the participants. Functioning levels, as used here, are usually classified as low, moderate, or high, or levels I, II, or III according to fitness performance. Instructors should look upon an adapted exercise or fitness activity as the medium through which objectives can be met. Cau-

---

[1]Claudine Sherrill, *Adapted Physical Education and Recreation*, 2nd ed. (Dubuque, Iowa: Wm. C. Brown, 1981), p. 95.
[2]*Ibid.*, pp. 96-97.

tion should be taken to ensure that the exercise or activity not be so modified, nor its challenges so diminished, that its benefits are destroyed. Adapted exercises and fitness activities may be used, where they are appropriate, in any of the programs described in the first section of this chapter.

No set procedures exist for adapting exercises or activities. The following guidelines may prove useful in making adaptations:

- Safety must be the prime consideration whenever adaptations are made.
- Adaptations should be made that permit disabled individuals to participate within the guidelines set forth by their physicians.
- Adaptations will be of no value if the individual is not motivated to participate.
- If capable, participants should be allowed input into the formulation of the adaptations in order to have a more positive attitude toward the adaptations and their utilization within exercises and activities.
- All adaptations or adjustments should be appropriate to the participant's physical status, chronological age, mental age, present performance level, and personal needs and interests.
- In some instances, only minor adjustments need be made that may allow the individual to perform the exercises and the activities.
- Whenever possible, the instructor should encourage the participant to use the regular methods and techniques to perform the exercises and the activities.

The following adaptations are organized under one or more of the fitness components, where appropriate, and examples are given of various types of handicapping conditions which may benefit from these suggested modifications. Many of the adaptations, however, may be made as a result of the instructor's innovativeness and resourcefulness.

CARDIOVASCULAR ENDURANCE

The following are suggested adaptations which assist in the development of cardiovascular endurance:

- Provide manual assistance when necessary.
- Provide music for walking and jogging to motivate participants.
- Provide crawling and creeping games for those unable to walk.
- Provide bicycle ergometers for those who cannot walk or jog.
- Provide for roller walkers or moon-buggies for those not capable of walking without devices.
- Provide low parallel bars for walking for the severely and profoundly retarded and others who need assistance.
- Provide a learning center for rolling, crawling, creeping, bouncing, and jumping rope.
- Use tires for bouncing.
- Measure and mark off in feet and yards an indoor course around a multi-purpose room or the gymnasium to accommodate crawling, creeping, walking, or jogging.
- Measure and mark off an outdoor walking or jogging course in fractions of miles and miles.
- Change jogging to walking, then to fast walking for participants who have heart problems, respiratory difficulties, and orthopedic handicaps.
- Run a lap and rest for a few seconds, run a lap and walk a lap, run a lap and ride a bike a lap, or run a lap and walk backward to starting position.
- Substitute rollerskating as a change from walking or jogging for those physically capable.
- Provide portable stairs for stepping up and down.
- Encourage the blind to hold the hand of a sighted participant or have each hold one end of a rolled towel for walking or jogging.
- Encourage the blind to hold on to a small piece of rope looped around a rope extended from post to post for walking or jogging.
- Offer rollerskating to the blind by using a sighted partner.
- Provide double runner skates for those who wish to learn to ice skate.
- Provide poles with miniature skis attached to the ends for leg amputee skiers.

- Change seats to chairs on bikes for better balance for those with cerebral palsy, deafness, and mental retardation.
- Weld two bikes together side-by-side for better balance for those with cerebral palsy, deafness, and mental retardation.
- Use a bicycle with two rear wheels to aid those learning to ride.
- Provide arm ergometers for paraplegics and those with cerebral palsy and others who cannot use bicycle ergometers.
- Provide rhythmic activities, folk and social dance for both enjoyment and elevation of the heart rate.
- When possible, provide all types of locomotor relay races, running and kicking a soccer or speedball, and line games such as soccer and basketball.
- Provide basketball dribbling relays, when possible, as a change from walking and jogging.
- Provide games using gym scooters for the non-ambulatory.
- Provide for wheelchair races: dashes, relay races, and distance races.
- Provide for wheelchair basketball, racquetball, and wallyball.
- Provide flotation aids for swimming, relay races, and water games.

MUSCULAR STRENGTH AND ENDURANCE

Listed below are adaptations which will assist in the development of muscular strength and endurance.

Weight-Training

- Provide manual assistance when necessary.
- Label the weights in braille for the blind or instruct them on how to find weight plates on the machine.
- Substitute sitting for the standing or military press.
- Attach a weight plate to the end of a rope and fasten it to a wooden dowel for performing wrist rolls.
- Provide a head harness attached to a wall pulley for neck exercises.
- Encourage paraplegics to perform the bench press by getting off the chair and on to the bench by themselves.

- Allow paraplegics to perform front raises, lateral raises, arm curls, tricep presses, and wrist rolls by holding the exercise bar with one hand.
- Instruct paraplegics to lean over the side of their chairs to perform arm curls with dumbbells.
- Assist paraplegics when they are performing the shoulder press or latissimus pulldown by pressing down on their shoulders and pressing against their chairs with one leg.
- Substitute logs for weights.
- Provide stuffed weighted animals for young children.
- Provide finger weights for those with weak finger muscles.
- Place the handle of a plastic pail containing sand on the top of the foot for performing leg extensions.
- Use medicine balls as weights.
- Place tires on and take them off a low portable standard.
- Provide elastic bandages for those with weak hand grips to secure the hands to the lever handles of the pulldown bar of the machine.
- Encourage a person with a single forearm amputation to wear a prosthesis in order to perform weight training exercises on a machine.

Timed Calisthenics

- Provide manual assistance when necessary.
- Provide exercises for any and all joints and body parts that have movement.
- Increase the time allowed to perform the exercise for beginners.
- Provide a rolled towel placed around the knees to assist in performing bent knee sit-ups.
- Provide a rolled towel placed around the toes to perform ankle flexion exercises.
- Encourage wheelchair bound participants to perform trunk bends with a twist by attempting to touch their chins to their thighs.
- Encourage wheelchair bound participants to perform chin-ups on an adjustable doorway gym bar placed against a door frame.

- Allow participants who wear braces or use crutches to change body positions to sitting or lying for performing exercises. Examples: leg raises, back raises, hip raises, straight leg sit-ups, straight leg trunk curls.
- Ask the participant with respiratory difficulties to start slowly and do breathing exercises while he/she assumes various body positions to improve his/her breathing patterns.
- Tell obese participants to start slowly and provide them with such exercises as push-ups, leg lifts, squat thrusts, straight leg sit-ups, and side sit-ups.
- Decrease the number of exercises within a specified time interval and provide a variety of exercises for the mentally retarded and emotionally disturbed because of their short attention span.

FLEXIBILITY

The following exercises will assist in the development of flexibility:

- Provide music while participants are exerising.
- Provide manual assistance when necessary.
- Manually guide the blind through each exercise until they learn from verbal commands.
- Demonstrate and provide visual aids and instructions for the deaf on how to perform each exercise.
- For the mentally retarded, provide a name for each exercise, explain how to perform each exercise in simple language, and demonstrate each exercise slowly.
- Encourage partner stretching when feasible.
- Encourage wheelchair-bound participants to perform sitting stretches predicated upon the severity of their handicap in their functional capacity.
- Provide exercise routines that focus upon all the joints and body parts.
- Progress slowly with each exercise until the participant's maximum range of motion at each joint is realized but give consideration to the participant's present physical status and potential.

- Provide a portable chin bar placed within a door frame for upper body stretching for the blind, the deaf, the mentally retarded, the emotionally disturbed, the one-arm amputee, and the wheelchair bound.
- Provide a rolled-up towel for upper body stretching.
- Change standing to sitting to perform stretching exercises.
- Change sitting to lying to perform stretching exercises.
- Provide portable stairs, a chair or bench for leg and hip stretches.
- Instruct participants not to bounce (ballistic stretching) in their attempt to increase their range of motion.
- Instruct participants to breath slowly and rhythmically while performing stretching exercises.
- Instruct participants to hold on to an exercise bar to perform waistline and arm and leg side stretches.

ADAPTED FITNESS PROGRAMS

Briefly described below are three adapted fitness programs.

Cardiac Rehabilitation

Cardiac Rehabilitation is an exercise program for people who have suffered a heart attack, have experienced open heart surgery, or may be significantly at risk of heart attacks. For these individuals, the advice and counsel of a cardiologist is essential in helping to develop the exercise prescription for the participant. Initially a treadmill stress test should be administered in a medical setting: in a hospital, a clinic, or a physician's office.

These types of exercise programs must have close medical supervision at each class session. The content for each class usually includes flexibility exercises and walking and/or slow jogging, and the class terminates with relaxation exercises. Sometimes a class session, which is forty-five minutes in length, may end with a volleyball game.

All participants must be referred to a cardiac exercise program by their personal physicians. While the progam provides

ongoing medical supervision during each exercise session, it is not
intended to replace the role of the primary physician. Throughout the program, periodic reports of progress should be provided
by the organization offering a cardiac rehabilitation exercise program.

Pulmonary Rehabilitation

Pulmonary Rehabilitation is an exercise program for individuals
who have asthma, chronic bronchitis, emphysema, or who otherwise
suffer from pulmonary insufficiency. Most of these types of programs are conducted in either hospitals or rehabilitation centers. As
with the cardiac exercise program, these participants must be referred to the pulmonary exercise program by their primary care
physician.

Pulmonary programs provide opportunities for individuals to receive instruction in the anatomy and physiology of respiration,
breathing exercises, relaxation exercises, respiratory hygiene, medications, and diets. The philosophy of a typical pulmonary rehabilitation exercise program is that learning should be active rather than
passive and that participants are part of an involved team and are
expected to share responsibility for their care. Classes and activities
should be planned and organized so as to provide individuals with
opportunities to learn and practice skills, integrate knowledge, and
become involved in personalizing their own home programs. The
instructor's major responsibility is to assess the participants' learning
needs, plan programs, guide participants' learning, and evaluate the
results.

Outdoor Fitness Courses
for the Disabled

A fitness course for disabled individuals can provide them with
a complete conditioning program. Such courses vary in length,
number of exercise stations, and degree of accessibility to persons with disabilities. Wheelchair fitness courses usually vary in
sophistication from circuits that are homemade to courses that are
produced   commercially.   Regardless   of   the   sophistication,

wheelchair fitness courses similar to a regular par course consist of warm-ups, muscular toning, cardiovascular endurance, and cool-down.*

---

*A manual may be purchased entitled *Fitness Courses with Adaptations for Persons Who are Disabled,* Vineland National Center, 3675 Ihduhapi Road, P.O. Box 308, Foretto, Minnesota 55357.

Note: Various forms which may help instructors in the development of fitness programs may be found in Appendices D to L.

APPENDICES

Appendix A
(Sample)

EXERCISE PRESCRIPTION

NAME: _____ Jane ----- _____ AGE: __ 14 __ HANDICAPPING CONDITION: __ Trainable Mentally Retarded __

Date _____

Height __ 4'10" __

Resting Heart Rate __ 72 __ Maximum Heart Rate __ 206 __ Training Heart Rate __ 164 __

Cardiovascular Evaluation __ Below average __ Results __ 50 yds. < __ Comments __ Interval training __

Weight __ 99 lbs. 45 kg __

Short Term Goal __ 50 yards __ Long Term Goal __ 300 yards __

Objectives	*Teaching Strategies*	*Evaluation of Performance*
		Completion Date
		Anticipated/Actual

Objectives

To enjoy exercise
To enhance competitive effort
To develop a habit

Teaching Strategies

Establish motivating criteria
Maximum output in short time
Keep exercises simple

Evaluation of Performance

Daily over the next 3 weeks
Completion in 12 weeks

General

Because of Jane's short interest span, instructor needs to motivate participant continuously. Avoid complex exercises and keep group small.

Exercise Recommendations

Use some warm-up stretches first
Train in 10-yard increments
Monitor heart rate response
End with some cool-down stretching

Specific

Exercise Style and Type:
   aerobic
Frequency: daily
Intensity: maximum output
   at shortest duration
Duration: to be determined
   by participant

Instructor's Name: _____

Adapted from *Fitness: A Lifetime Commitment* by David K. Miller and T. Earl Allen, p. 187, 2nd ed., 1982, Burgess Publishing Company, Minneapolis, Minnesota.

147

Appendix A (continued)

Date _____

Height _____ 5'8"

Weight _____ 149.6 lbs. 68 kg

(Sample)

EXERCISE PRESCRIPTION

NAME: ___ James ----- ___ AGE: ___ 25 ___ HANDICAPPING CONDITION: ___ Paraplegic

Resting Heart Rate ___ 75 ___ Maximum Heart Rate ___ 195 ___ Training Heart Rate ___ 164

Cardiovascular Evaluation ___ Below average ___ Results ___ 8 mets* ___ Comments ___ Arm ergometer

Short Term Goal: ___ Improve upper body strength ___ Long Term Goal ___ Improve cardiovascular fitness

Objectives	*Teaching Strategies*	*Evaluation of Performance* *Completion Date* *Anticipated/Actual*
Improve flexibility	Stretching exercises, 10-15 min.	Completion in 10 weeks
Improve strength	Weight training, 20-30 min.	Begin Program
Improve cardiovascular fitness	Arm ergometer, 20 min.	

General	*Exercise Recommendations*	*Specific*
Weight training program with aerobic component	Arm ergometer	Exercise Style and Type: aerobic Frequency: 3x weekly Intensity: THR** of 164 bpm*** Duration: goal of 20 min.

Instructor's Name: _____

*One met is equal to 3.5 milliliters per kilogram per minute

**target heart rate

***beats per minute

Appendix A (continued)

(Sample)

EXERCISE PRESCRIPTION

Date _____

NAME: ___ Joe ----- ___ AGE: __40__ HANDICAPPING CONDITION: __Coronary artery disease__

Height __5'10"__

Resting Heart Rate __60__ Maximum Heart Rate __124__ Training Heart Rate __104__

Weight __176 lbs. 80 kg__

Cardiovascular Evaluation __Below average__ Results __7.5 mets__ Comments __Medicated — Beta Blocker__

Short Term Goal __Abdominal toning__ Long Term Goal __Improve cardiovascular fitness__

Evaluation of Performance
Completion Date
Anticipated/Actual

Objectives	*Teaching Strategies*	
Improve flexibility	Slow stretching exercises, 10-15 min.	Completion in 10 weeks
Increase abdominal strength	Progressive curl-ups and let-downs, etc., 10 min	Begin program
Improve cardiovascular fitness	Brisk walking or jogging, 20 min.	

General	*Exercise Recommendations*	*Specific*
Monitored calisthenics	Swimming	Exercise Style and Type: aerobic
and jogging at suggested	Jogging	Frequency: 3x weekly
THR of 104 bpm for 10 weeks	Bike ergometer	Intensity: THR of 104 bpm
		Duration: goal of 20 min.

Instructor's Name: _____

Appendix A (continued)

(Sample)

EXERCISE PRESCRIPTION

Date _____

Height _____ 5'2"

Weight _____ 110 lbs. 50 kg

NAME: _____ Mary ----- _____ AGE: _____ 65 _____ HANDICAPPING CONDITION: _____ Emphysema

Resting Heart Rate _____ 80 _____ Maximum Heart Rate _____ 140 _____ Training Heart Rate _____ 120

Cardiovascular Evaluation _____ Below average _____ Results _____ 3.5 mets _____ Comments _____ Respiratory medication in use

Short Term Goal _____ Improve range of motion _____ Long Term Goal _____ Improve cardiovascular fitness

Objectives   *Teaching Strategies*   *Evaluation of Performance*
Completion Date
Anticipated/Actual

Increase flexibility   Slow stretching exercises   Completion in 6 months

Increase strength   Mild resistance exercises   Begin program _____

Improve pulmonary function   Diaphragmatic breathing

General   *Exercise Recommendations*   *Specific*

Monitored calisthenics   Walking   Exercise Style and Type:

Brisk walking and bike   Bike ergometer   aerobic

ergometer for 6 months   Frequency: 3x weekly

                                         Intensity: THR of 120 bpm

                                         Duration: goal of 20 min.

Instructor's Name: _____

MUSCULAR STRENGTH AND
ENDURANCE PROGRAM CONTRACT

Participant's Name _____ Grade Level _____ Age _____

Handicapping Condition _____

Present Fitness Status; _____ Poor _____ Good _____ Very Good _____ Weight _____ Excellent

Rest Periods; _____ 1 minute _____ 2 minutes of alternating exercises

WEIGHT TRAINING

WEEK	DAYS	BODY PARTS	TYPE OF EXERCISE	SETS	REPETITIONS	RESISTANCE	COMMENTS
1							
2							
3							
4							
5							
6							
7							

Appendix B (continued)

WEEK	DAYS	BODY PARTS	TYPE OF EXERCISE	SETS	REPETITIONS	RESISTANCE	COMMENTS
8							
9							
10							
11							
12							

Participant's signature _____

Contract approval date _____

Contract completion date _____

Reason contract was terminated _____

Date contract was terminated _____

Instructor's signature _____

Appendix B (continued)

CARDIOVASCULAR ENDURANCE PROGRAM CONTRACT

Participant's Name _____   Grade Level _____   Age _____

Handicapping Condition _____

Present Fitness Status; _____ Poor _____ Good _____ Very Good _____ Weight _____ Excellent

Type of Cardiovascular Exercise(s); _____ Walking _____ Jogging _____ Jump Rope _____ Treadmill

_____ Stationary Bike _____ Arm ergometer _____ Aerobic Rebound Exerciser

Recommended Exercise Heart Rate _____

WEEK	DAYS	EXERCISE	HEART RATE	DURATION	COMMENTS
1					
2					
3					
4					
5					
6					
7					

Appendix B (continued)

WEEK	DAYS	EXERCISE	HEART RATE	DURATION	COMMENTS
8					
9					
10					

Participant's signature _____

Contract approval date _____

Contract completion date _____

Reason contract was terminated _____

Date contract was terminated _____

Instructor's signature _____

TIMED CALISTHENICS PROGRAM CONTRACT

Participant's Name _____ Grade Level _____ Age _____

Handicapping Condition _____ Weight _____

Present Fitness Status; _____ Poor _____ Good _____ Very Good _____ Excellent

Rest Periods; _____ minutes _____ minutes

BODY PARTS	TYPE OF EXERCISE	SETS	REPETITIONS	COMMENTS

Participant's signature _____

Contract approval date _____

Contract completion date _____

Reason contract was terminated _____

Date contract was terminated _____

Instructor's signature _____

Appendix B (continued)

FLEXIBILITY PROGRAM CONTRACT

Participant's Name _____ Grade Level _____ Age _____

Handicapping Condition _____

Present Fitness Status; _____ Poor _____ Good _____ Very Good _____ Excellent

Rest Periods; _____ minutes _____ minutes

Weight _____

BODY PARTS	TYPE OF EXERCISE	SETS	REPETITIONS	COMMENTS

Participant's signature _____

Contract approval date _____

Contract completion date _____

Reason contract was terminated _____

Date contract was terminated _____

Instructor's signature _____

Appendix C

SUGGESTED LISTING OF PHYSICAL FITNESS ACTIVITIES CLASSIFIED BY MAJOR COMPONENT PROVIDED FOR THE INSTRUCTOR

Activities Should be Selected According to Ages, Handicapping Conditions and Functioning Levels of the Participants

CARDIOVASCULAR ENDURANCE

*Aquatic Games
  Ball Tag
  Dodge Ball
  Fish and Net
  Follow the Leader
  Keep Away
  Walking Race
Arm Ergometer
Badminton
Bicycle Ergometer
Bicycling
Bouncing on Trampoline
Climbing Stairs

*Dances
  Aerobic
  Folk
  Rhythmics
  Singing Games
  Social
  Square
Dribbling Balls with Hands or Feet
Field Hockey
Football
Gym Scooter Activities
Handball
Hiking

---

*Denotes a group of physical fitness activities. Methods for teaching them may be found in most elementary physical education books.

157

Indoor Fitness Course

Jogging

Jumping Rope

Lacrosse

*Line Games

  Basketball

  Dodge Ball

  Floor Hockey

*Locomotor Movements

  Crawling

  Creeping

  Galloping

  Hopping

  Jumping

  Leaping

  Running

  Skipping

  Sliding

  Walking

Marching

Mountain Climbing

Moving Feet to Propel a
  Wheelchair

Outdoor Fitness Course

Racquetball

*Relay Races

  Baton Passing

  Crows and Cranes

  Gym Scooter

  Indian Club

  Jump Rope

  Line

  Pilot

  Pin

  Pushing a Moon Buggy

  Sack

  Wheelchair

Skating (Ice and Roller)

Skiing (Cross Country)

Snowshoeing

Squash

Swimming

Table Tennis

*Tag Games

  Bear in the Pit

  Capture the Flag

  Cat and Mouse

  Chain

  Circle Run

  Cross Tag

  Man from Mars

  Pom-Pom Pullaway

  Rabbits and Foxes

  Scooter

  Steal the Bacon

Tennis

Treadmill

Tricyling

Volleyball

Walking

Wheelchair Soccer

---

*Denotes a group of physical fitness activities. Methods for teaching them may be found in most elementary physical education books.

MUSCULAR STRENGTH

Archery

Arm Travel on Parallel Bars

Climbing Ropes

Exercises Using Inner Tube Strips

Gymnastics

Hang from Chinning Bar or Horizontal Ladder

*Isometrics (Create other exercises to include other muscle groups and body parts. Hold all exercises for six to eight-second counts.)

Bend knees and press against the wall
Lock fingers, place behind neck and press backward
Lock fingers, place on forehead and press forward
Press back to back with a partner
Press feet to feet with a partner
Press hand to hand with a partner
Press a ball against the floor
Press buttocks against wall
Press feet against wall
Press shoulders against wall
Press forehead against wall
Pull a towel or rope horizontally
Squeeze ball between hands
Squeeze ball between legs
Squeeze ball in one hand
Step on towel or rope, holding onto both ends, arms bent, pull
Step on towel or rope, holding onto both ends, arms extended, pull

King of the Hill

Medicine Ball Exercises
Rowing

---

*These exercises are briefly described.

*Stunts
  Carry Partner on Shoulders
  Chinese Stand-Up
  Cock Fight
  Elephant Walk
  Hand and Indian Wrestling
  Leap Frog
  Lift Partner Up
  Rocker
  Pull Across
  Wheelbarrel
Timed Calisthenics
Weight Training
  Barbells
  Bricks
  Dumbbells
  Logs
  Machines
  Sandbags
  Socks Filled With Sand
  Stuffed Animals
Wrestling

**MUSCULAR ENDURANCE

Aqua-Dynamic Exercises
Basketball
Bouncing on Trampoline
Canoeing
Cycling
Gymnastics
Hiking
Isometrics
Jogging
Jumping Rope

Marching
Obstacle Course
Skating (Roller and Ice)
Soccer
Swimming
Timed Calisthenics
Volleyball
Walking
Weight Training

---

*Denotes a group of physical fitness activities. Methods for teaching them may be found in most elementary physical education books.
**Refer to cardiovascular endurance for other muscular endurance activities.

FLEXIBILITY

Arm Raisers

Bird Flying

Bend at Hips — forward, backward and to the sides

Body Movements while in a wheelchair (also done to music)

Body Twists to Music

Circles — with head, hands, arms, legs, and feet

Dry Land Swimming

Grapevine

Move ankle joints

Move hips and vertebral joints

Move knee joints

Move shoulder joints

Rocker

Sit-up — touch toes

Stand — touch toes with knees straight

Stand — touch heels

V-sit

*Non-Locomotor Movements

   Stretching and Bending
   Swaying and Swinging
   Turning and Twisting

---

*Denotes a group of physical fitness activities. Methods for teaching them may be found in most elementary physical education books.

Appendix D

PHYSICAL ACTIVITY PROFILE

NAME _____   DATE _____

Please answer the following questions about your job and non-job related physical activity.

1) **IN WHAT KIND OF BUSINESS OR INDUSTRY DO YOU WORK:** (for example, electronics manufacturing, insurance company, food store)

FIRM_____   POSITION_____

2) HOW WOULD YOU RATE THE INTENSITY OF PHYSICAL ACTIVITY YOU PERFORM AT WORK?

very little	little	moderate	active	very active
/	/	/	/	/

3) HOW WOULD YOU RATE THE INTENSITY OF PHYSICAL ACTIVITY YOU PERFORM DURING YOUR LEISURE TIME?

very little	little	moderate	active	very active
/	/	/	/	/

4) WHAT PHYSICAL ACTIVITIES, IF ANY, ARE YOU PRESENTLY PARTICIPATING IN?

_____

5) DURING THE PAST TWO YEARS, HAVE YOU STARTED ANY NEW PHYSICAL ACTIVITIES WHICH HAVE SINCE BEEN DISCONTINUED?_____

_____

6) HOW WOULD YOU BEST DESCRIBE YOUR PRESENT LEVEL OF FITNESS?

poor	fair	average	good	excellent
/	/	/	/	/

7) PROVIDING THE EQUIPMENT AND FACILITIES WERE AVAILABLE, IN WHICH PHYSICAL ACTIVITIES WOULD YOU BE INTERESTED IN LEARNING AND PARTICIPATING? PLEASE CHECK OR LIST ACTIVITIES.

Rowing_____ Tennis_____ Mt. Climbing_____
Jogging_____ Racquetball_____ Weight Training_____
Bicycling_____ Volleyball_____ Hiking_____
Swimming_____ Canoeing_____ Cross Country Skiing____
Orienteering_____ Other (specify_____

8) DO YOU HAVE ANY EXERCISE EQUIPMENT OR DEVICE AT HOME?
YES _____   NO _____

(Pool, stationary bike, weights, etc., please list) _____

Source: Lawrence A. Golding, Clayton R. Myers, and Wayne E. Sinning, editors, *The Y's Way to Physical Fitness*, YMCA of the USA, Program Resources, 6400 Shafter Court, Rosemont, IL 60018, (Revised, 1982).

Appendix E

GENERAL MEDICAL HISTORY

(To be completed by the participant, if possible. If not, the instructor.)

NAME _____ TEL. _____ DATE _____

STREET _____ CITY _____ ZIP _____ AGE _____

Circle One

Any medical complaints? _____ YES   NO

_____

_____

Any major illness in past? (Give dates) _____ YES   NO

_____

_____

Any hospitalization? _____ YES   NO

_____

_____

Smoke now? _____   Packages per day _____ YES   NO

Smoked in past? _____   Packages per day _____ YES   NO

Weight gain in past ten years _____ lbs.

Weight at age   20 _____   30 _____   40 _____   50 _____

Diabetes? _____ YES   NO

Family history of diabetes? _____ Who? _____ YES NO

Family history of heart disease? _____ Who?_____ YES NO

Family history of high blood pressure?_____ Who? _____ YES NO

Family history of muscular illness? _____ Who? _____ YES NO

Please list any present medications/drugs you are taking _____

CARDIORESPIRATORY HISTORY

Any heart disease now?	YES	NO	Daily coughing?	YES	NO
Any heart disease in past?	YES	NO	Cough produces sputum?	YES	NO
Heart murmers?	YES	NO	High blood pressure?	YES	NO
Occasional chest pains	YES	NO	Shortness of breath at rest?	YES	NO
			Shortness of breath after two flights of stairs?	YES	NO

MUSCULAR HISTORY

Any muscle injuries or illness now?	YES	NO	Muscular weakness now?	YES	NO
			Muscular illness now?	YES	NO
Any muscular injuries or illness in past?	YES	NO	Muscle pain at rest?	YES	NO
			Muscle pain at exertion?	YES	NO

BONE JOINT HISTORY

Any bone or joint (including spine) injuries or illnesses now?	YES	NO	Ever had swollen joints?	YES	NO
			Ever had painful joints?	YES	NO
			Flat feet?	YES	NO
Any bone or joint (including spine) injuries or illnesses in past?	YES	NO	Allergies?	YES	NO
			Specify _____	YES	NO

COMMENTS: _____

Source: Lawrence A. Golding, Clayton R. Myers, and Wayne E. Sinning, editors *The Y's Way to Physical Fitness,* YMCA of the USA, Program Resources, 6400 Shafter Court, Rosemont, IL 60018. (Revised, 1982)

Appendix F
INFORMED CONSENT FORM

In consideration of being accepted into this program, I do, on behalf of myself and my heirs or executor release and discharge the organization, the institution and/or school and all its agents from any claims or demands which I may have now or at any time in the future resulting from any illnesses on injurious occurrences as a result of participation in this program.

The assessment includes the following tests: (1) Cardiorespiratory fitness, (2) body composition, (3) flexibility, and (4) muscular strength and endurance. The most physically demanding test is that of cardiorespiratory fitness.

The cardiorespiratory fitness test consists of riding on a specially-designed bicycle or walking/running on an exercise treadmill. The purpose is to examine your heart rate response to submaximal exercise and recovery periods.

Complications have been few during exercise tests, especially those of submaximal nature. If the person exercising is not tolerating work well, it usually becomes apparent and the exercise is stopped. Mild lightheadedness and even fainting may occur but they are not usual and disappear quickly on lying down. Other risks of injury while climbing onto or off the bicycle/or treadmill are possible but are rare.

In signing this consent form, you state that you have read and understood the description of the tests and their complications. Any questions which occur to you have been answered to your satisfaction. Every effort will be exerted to insure your health and safety.

You enter into the tests willingly and may withdraw at any time.

The information which is obtained during the laboratory evaluations and exercise sessions of the fitness program will be treated as privileged and confidential and will not be released or revealed to any non-medical person without your expressed written consent. The information obtained, however, may be used for a statistical or scientific purpose with your right of privacy retained. You also approve of periodic forwarding to your physician of data relative to your laboratory evaluations and exercise sessions.

Furthermore, you agree to look to your private physician for medical care as he deems necessary.

_____   _____
(Print name of family physician)   (Address of family physician)

_____   _____
Signature of applicant   (Date)

Source: Lawrence A. Golding, Clayton R. Myers, and Wayne E. Sinning, editors, *The Y's Way to Physical Fitness,* YMCA of the USA, Program Resources, 6400 Shafter Court, Rosemont, IL 60018 (Revised, 1982).

Appendix G

GRADED EXERCISE TEST

DATE:_____ NAME:_____ AGE:_____

MEDICATIONS:_____

REFERRING PHYSICIAN:_____ PROTOCOL:_____

ATTENDING PHYSICIAN:_____ TECHNICIAN:_____

****

STAGE	RPE	RATE	BP	ST SEGMENT	ARRHYTHMIA	SYMPTOMS - CODE
SUPINE						0-NONE
STANDING						1-CHEST PAIN
POST-HYPER						2-MILD DYSPNEA
S-I						3-MOD. DYSPNEA
						4-SEVERE DYSPNEA
						5-GEN. FATIGUE

Appendix G (continued)

STAGE	RPE	RATE	BP	ST SEGMENT	ARRHYTHMIA	SYMPTOMS - CODE
						6-LEG FATIGUE
						7-CLAUDICATION
						8-DIZZINESS
						9-FAINTNESS
						10-HYPOTENSIVE
						11-OTHER

TOTAL TIME[3] _____ min.   PEAK MET LEVEL[3] _____   SPB X HR/100[3] _____

PREDICTED MAX. HR[3] _____   85% PMHR[3] _____   ATTAINED HR[3] _____   % PMHR[3] _____

85% FWC_____MIN.   02 UPTAKE_____ML/KG/MIN.   CV LEVEL_____   % THR_____ TO_____ BPM
                                                                    THR_____ TO_____ 15 Sec

****

INTERPRETATION:

Source: University of Southern Maine's Adult Fitness Programs — Lifeline.

Appendix H

PHYSICIAN REFERRAL FORM

CARDIAC REHABILITATION PROGRAM

Patient's Name _____ Date _____

Last   First   Initial

Address _____ Age _____ Phone _____

I consider the above individual as:

_____ Cardiac Patient

_____ Prone to Coronary Heart Disease

_____ Other (explain) _____

NOTE: Primary risk factors are hypertension, hyperlipidemia, and cigarette smoking. Secondary risk factors are family history, obesity, physical inactivity, diabetes mellitus and asymptomatic hyperglycemia.

Diagnostic Data
Etiologic

1. No heart disease
2. Rheumatic
3. Congenital
4. Hypertension
5. CAD
6. Other

Present
Physical Activity

1. Very active
2. Normal
3. Limited
4. Very limited

EKG

1. Normal
2. Dig. effect only
3. Other abnormalities-specify
4. Infarct

Rhythm

1. Sinus
2. Atrial Fib.
3. Other

Specific cardiac diagnosis _____

Additional abnormalities you are aware of _____

_____

170

Appendix H (continued)

Date of last complete physical examination_____

Present medication_____

Please fill in the information below if it is available:

1. Urine, sp. gr._____ Alb._____ Glucose_____ Micro._____

2. Complete blood count: Hbg._____ Hct._____ WBC_____ Diff._____

3. ECG, 12 lead (enclose copy)_____

4. Blood pressure, syst._____ Diast._____

5. Cholesterol_____mg% 2 hr. post prandial_____ Triglyceride_____mg%.

6. Masters, and/or Graded Exercise Test Results (if available, enclose)_____

Impression of above information_____

_____

The above-listed person is capable of participating in a mild exercise program, as well as periodic laboratory evaluations, under the guidance of a competent, well-trained physical educator and supervision of a physician.

Signed:_____, M.D.

Type or Print
Name of Physician_____

Address_____ Tel._____

Adapted from *Policies and Procedures of a Cardiac Rehabilitation Program: Immediate to Long-Term Care* by P. K. Wilson, E. R. Winga, J. W. Edgett and T. T. Gushiken. Lea & Febiger, 1978.

Appendix I

CARDIAC REHABILITATION PROGRAM
INFORMED CONSENT FORM

I desire to engage voluntarily in the Cardiac Rehabilitation Program for guidance and supervision in safe exercise. My participation in this program has been recommended and approved by my physician, Dr._____.

Before I enter the exercise phase of the program, I will have a clinical evaluation. This evaluation will include **medical history** of heart rate and blood pressure, EKG at rest and during exercise. The exercise test will consist of walking on a treadmill at varying levels of speed and grade. This increase in effort will continue until a predetermined heart rate response is achieved or adverse symptoms preclude continuation. During the performance of the test, a physician and trained observers will monitor my pulse, blood pressure, and electrocardiogram. There exists the possibility of certain changes occurring during the exercise test. They include abnormal blood pressure or pulse rate and very rare instances of "heart attack." The purpose of this evaluation is to detect any condition which would indicate that I should not engage in this exercise program and to determine the level of exercise for me during the three-per-week exercise sessions. The exercise sessions will allow personalized exercise levels based upon the graded exercise test evaluation and will be carefully regulated by the supervisor of the exercise program. The exercise activities are designed to place a gradually increasing workload on the cardiovascular system. The reaction of the cardiovascular system to such activities cannot always be predicted with complete accuracy.

Therefore, there is the risk of abnormal blood pressure or pulse rate and, in rare instances, "heart attack" occurring during or following the exercise.

Before initially participating in the exercise phase of the Cardiac Rehabilitation Program, I will be instructed as to the signs and symptoms which I should report promptly to the supervisor of the exercises. I also will be observed by the supervisor of the exercises, or an assigned assistant, who will be alert to changes which would suggest that I modify my exercise. Emergency equipment and trained personnel are available to deal with and minimize the dangers of untoward events should they occur.

This information which is obtained during the laboratory evaluations and exercise sessions of the Cardiac Rehabilitation Program will be treated as privileged and confidential and will not be released or revealed to any non-medical person without my expressed written consent. The information obtained, however, may be used for a statistical or scientific purpose with my right of privacy retained. I also approve of periodic forwarding to and from my physician of any **medical records** relative to my laboratory evaluations and exercise sessions.

I have read the foregoing, and I understand it. Any questions which have arisen or occurred to me have been answered to my satisfaction.

Signed:

_____   _____

Patient   Physician

_____

Date

Adapted from *Policies and Procedures of a Cardiac Rehabilitation Program: Immediate to Long-Term Care* by P. K. Wilson, E. R. Winga, J. W. Edgett and T. T. Gushiken, Lea & Febiger, 1978.

Appendix J

CARDIAC REHABILITATION PROGRAM
Exercise Session Daily Data Sheet

Name_____Age_____B/P_____THR_____

Medications_____

Primary
Physician_____Cardiologist_____

Diagnosis: Post MI_____, CABG_____, CAD_____, Diabetic_____

Other_____

DATE							
Weight							
Entering B/P							
Entering H/R							
C.V. #1 HR							

Appendix J (continued)

C. V. #2 HR						
C. V. #3 HR						
Cool Down HR						
2 Min. Post Ex HR						
2 Min. Post Ex B/P						
Remarks						

Source: University of Southern Maine's Adult Fitness Programs — Lifeline.

Appendix K
PULMONARY INFORMED
CONSENT FORM

In consideration of being accepted into this program, I do, on behalf of myself and my heirs or executor release and discharge the organization, institution and/or the school and all its agents from any claims or demands which I may have now or at any time in the future resulting from any illnesses or injurious occurrences as a result of participation in this program.

Periodic pulmonary function tests may be required to ascertain respiratory fitness. Although this is a relatively safe method of evaluation, induction of some coughing, wheezing, lightheadedness and pulmonary spasm is possible.

Exercises which are designed to improve breathing may also produce these symptoms.

All tests and exercises will be done with your health and safety in mind by well trained fitness instructors.

In signing this consent form, you state that you have read and understood the description of the tests and their complications. Any questions which occur to you have been answered to your satisfaction. Every effort will be exerted to insure your health and safety. You enter into the tests willingly and may withdraw at any time.

The information which is obtained during the laboratory evaluations and exercise sessions of the pulmonary program will be treated as privileged and confidential and will not be released or revealed to any non-medical person without your expressed written consent. The information obtained, however, may be used for a statistical or scientific purpose with your right of privacy retained. You also approve of periodic forwarding to your physician of data relative to your laboratory evaluations and exercise sessions.

Futhermore, you agree to look to your private physician for medical care and agree to have an evaluation by him at least once a year.

_____ _____

(Print name of family physician) (Address of family physician)

_____ _____

(Signature of Applicant)   (Date)

Source: University of Southern Maine's Adult Fitness Programs-Lifeline.

Appendix L

PULMONARY EXERCISE RECORD

NAME _____ TARGET HR _____ AGE _____ DIAGNOSIS _____

PHYSICIAN _____ STRESS TEST _____ MEDS _____

DATE																
RESTING BLOOD PRESSURE																
RESTING HEART RATE																
POST WARM-UP HEART RATE																

Appendix L (continued)

C.V. #1 HR																
C.V. #2 HR																
C.V. #3 HR																
# OF MINUTES																
POST COOL-DOWN HEARTRATE																
POST COOL-DOWN BLOOD PRESSURE																

COMMENTS:

Source: University of Southern Maine's Adult Fitness Programs — Lifeline.

BIBLIOGRAPHY

1. Allsen, Philip E.: *Conditioning and Physical Fitness: Current Answers to Relevant Questions.* Dubuque, Brown, 1978.
2. Allsen, Philip E., Harrison, Joyce M., and Vance, Barbara: *Fitness for Life: An Individualized Approach,* 2nd ed. Dubuque, Brown, 1980.
3. American Alliance for Health, Physical Education and Recreation: *Annotated Research Bibliography in Physical Education, Recreation and Psychomotor Function of Mentally Retarded Persons.* Washington, D.C., AAHPER, 1975.
4. American Alliance for Health, Physical Education and Recreation: *Special Fitness Test Manual for Mildly Mentally Retarded Persons.* Washington, D.C., AAHPER — Kennedy Foundation, 1976.
5. American Alliance for Health, Physical Education, Recreation and Dance: *Health Related Physical Fitness Test Manual.* Reston, VA, AAHPERD, 1980.
6. American Alliance for Health, Physical Education, Recreation and Dance: *Health Related Physical Fitness Test Technical Manual.* Reston, VA, AAHPERD, 1984.
7. American Association for Health, Physical Education and Recreation: *Physical Education and Recreation for the Visually Handicapped.* Washington, D.C., AAHPER, 1973.
8. American College of Sports Medicine: *Guidelines for Graded Exercise Testing and Exercise Prescription,* 2nd ed. Philadelphia, Lea & Febiger, 1980.
9. American Heart Association: Committee on Exercise: *Exercise Testing and Training of Individuals with Heart Disease or a High Risk for its Development: A Handbook for Physicians.* Dallas, American Heart Association, 1975.
10. American National Red Cross: *Adapted Aquatics: Swimming for Persons with Physical or Mental Impairments.* Garden City, Doubleday, 1977.
11. Anderson, Bob: *Stretching.* Bolinas, CA, Shelter Pub., 1980.
12. Asrtrand, Per-Olof and Saltin, Bengt: Maximal oxygen uptake and heart rate in various types of muscular activity. *J Appl Physiol, 16*:977-981, 1961.
13. Barach, Alvan L., and Petty, Thomas L.: Is chronic obstructive lung disease improved by physical exercise? (Editorial). *JAMA, 234*:854-855, 1975.

14. Basmajian, John V.: *Therapeutic Exercise,* 4th ed. Baltimore, Williams and Wilkins, 1984.
15. Bauer, Dan: Aerobic fitness for the moderately retarded. *Practical Pointers, 5,* November 1981.
16. Bauer, Dan: Aerobic fitness for the severely and profoundly mentally retarded. *Practical Pointers, 5,* November 1981.
17. Berg, Kristina: Effect of physical training of school children with cerebral palsy. *Acta Paediatrica Scandinavica, 204*:27-33, 1970.
18. Berg, Kristina; Remarks on physical training of children with cerebral palsy. *Acta Paediatrica Scandinavica Suppl., 217*:106-107, 1971.
19. Berg, Kristina and Isaksson, Bjorn: Body composition and nutrition of school children with cerebral palsy. *Acta Paediatrica Scandinavica, 204*:41-52, 1970.
20. Berg, Kristina and Bjure, Jan: Methods for evaluation of the physical working capacity of school children with cerebral palsy. *Acta Paediatrica Scandinavica, 204*:15-26, 1970.
21. Bevegard, Sture, Freyschuss, Ulla, and Strandell, Tore: Circulatory adaptation to arm and leg exercise in supine and sitting position. *J Appl Physiol, 21*:37-46, 1966.
22. Brown, Alan: Review: Physical fitness and cerebral palsy. *Child: Care, Health and Development, 1*:143-152, 1975.
23. Brown, Jeannette A., and Pate, Robert H., Jr.: *Being A Counselor: Directions and Challenges.* Monterey, Brooks/Cole, 1983.
24. Buell, Charles E.: *Physical Education and Recreation for the Visually Handicapped,* Rev. ed. Reston, VA, AAHPERD, 1982.
25. Buell, Charles E: *Physical Education for Blind Children*, 2nd ed. Springfield, Thomas, 1983.
26. Burke, Edmund J.: *Exercise, Science and Fitness.* Ithaca, Mouvement Pubns., 1980.
27. Campbell, Jack: Physical Fitness and the MR: A review of research. *Mental Retardation, 11(5)*:26-29, Oct., 1973.
28. Case, Samuel, Dawson, Yvette, Schartner, James, Donaway, Dale: Comparison of levels of fundamental skill and cardio-respiratory fitness of blind, deaf, and non-handicapped high school age boys. *Perceptual and Motor Skills, 36*:1291-1294, 1973.
29. Cautela, Joseph R. and Groden, June: *Relaxation: A Comprehensive Manual for Adults, Children, and Children with Special Needs.* Champaign, IL, Research Press, 1978.
30. Chawla, J. C., Bar, C., Creber, I., Price, J., and Andrews, B.: Techniques for improving the strength and fitness of spinal injured patients. *Paraplegia, 17(2)*:185-189, July, 1979.
31. Cooper, Kenneth H.: *The Aerobics Program for Total Well-Being.* New York, M. Evans, 1982.
32. Cooper, Kenneth H.: *The New Aerobics.* New York, Bantam Books, 1970.
33. Cooper, Mildred, and Cooper, Kenneth H.: *Aerobics for Women.* New York, Bantam Books, 1972.

34. Corbin, Charles B. and Lindsey, Ruth: *Fitness for Life,* 2nd ed. Glenview, IL, Scott, Foresman, 1983.

35. Corder, W. Owen: Effects of physical education on the intellectual, physical, and social development of educable mentally retarded boys. *Exceptional Children, 32*:357-364, 1966.

36. Cratty, Bryant J.: *Adapted Physical Education for Handicapped Children and Youth.* Denver, Love Pub., 1980.

37. Crowe, Walter C., Auxter, David, and Pyfer, Jean: *Principles and Methods of Adapted Physical Education and Recreation,* 4th ed. St. Louis, Mosby, 1981.

38. Daniels, Lucille, and Worthingham, Catherine: *Therapeutic Exercise for Body Alignment and Function,* 2nd ed. Philadelphia, Saunders, 1977.

39. Danielson, Richard R., and Danielson, Karen F., editors: *Fitness Motivation.* Toronto, Orcol Pubns., 1980.

40. Davis, Glen M., Kofsky, Peggy R., Kelsey, Janice C., Shephard, Roy J.: Cardiorespiratory fitness and muscular strength of wheelchair users. *CMA Journal, 125*:1317-1323, 1981.

41. Delza, Sophia: *Body and Mind in Harmony.* New York, McKay, 1961.

42. Descoeudres, Alice: *The Education of Mentally Defective Children.* Boston, Heath, 1928.

43. Effgen, Susan K.: Effect of an exercise program on the static balance of deaf children. *Physical Therapy, 61*:873-877, 1981.

44. Ekblom, Bjorn and Lundberg, Ake: Effect of physical training on adolescents with severe motor handicaps. *Acta Paediatrica Scandinavica, 57*:17-23, 1968.

45. Emes, Claudia G.: Fitness and the physically disabled — a review. *Canadian Journal of Applied Sport Sciences, 6(4)*:176-178, December, 1981.

46. Emes, Claudia G.: Maintenance of uncued isometric contractions by blind and sighted. *Perceptual and Motor Skills, 49*:475-479, 1979.

47. Fait, Hollis F. and Dunn, John M.: *Special Physical Education: Adapted, Individualized and Developmental,* 5th ed. Philadelphia, Saunders, 1983.

48. Falls, Harold B.: Modern concepts of physical fitness. *Journal of Physical Education and Recreation, 51(4)*:25-27, April 1980.

49. Falls, Harold B., Baylor, Ann M. and Dishman, Rod K.: *Essentials of Fitness.* Philadelphia, Saunders College, 1980.

50. Fitch, Kenneth D.: Comparative aspects of available exercise systems. *Pediatrics, 56*:904-907, 1975.

51. Fitch, K. D. and Morton, A. R.: Specificity of exercise in exercise-induced asthma. *British Medical Journal, 4*:577-581, 1971.

52. Fitch, K. D., Morton, A. R., and Blanksby, B. A.: Effects of swimming training on children with asthma. *Archives of Diseases in Childhood, 51*:190-194, 1976.

53. Fox, Edward L., Mathews, Donald K. and Barstow, Jeffrey N.: *I.T.: Interval Training for Lifetime Fitness.* New York, Dial, 1980.

54. Gentz, J., Hamfelt, A., Johansson, S., Lindstedt, S., Persson, B. and Zetterstrom, R.: Vitamin B_6 metabolism in pyridoxine dependence with seizures. *Acta Paediatrica Scandinavica, 56*:17-26, 1967.

55. Getchell, Bud: *Physical Fitness: A Way of Life,* 3rd ed. New York, Wiley, 1983.
56. Ghory, Joseph R.: Exercise and asthma: overview and clinical impact. *Pediatrics, 56:*844-860, 1975.
57. Godfrey, Simon: *Exercise Testing in Children.* London, Saunders, 1974.
58. Golding, Lawrence A., Myers, Clayton R. and Sinning, Wayne E.: *The Y's Way to Physical Fitness.* Chicago, National Board of YMCA, 1982.
59. Hayden, Frank J.: *Physical Fitness for the Mentally Retarded — A Manual for Teachers and Parents.* Toronto, Metropolitan Toronto Association for Retarded Children, 1964.
60. Healey, Alfred: Two methods of weight-training for children with spastic type of cerebral palsy. *Research Quarterly, 29:*389-395, 1958.
61. Hershfield, Sherman, Kottke, Frederic J., Kubicek, William G., Olson, Mildred E., Boen, James, Lillquist, Cecelia, and Stradal, Larry: Relative effects on the heart by muscular work in the upper and lower extremities. *Arch Phys Med Rehabil, 49(5):*249-257, May 1968.
62. Heyes, Anthony David: Blindness and yoga. *The New Outlook, 68(9):*385-393, November 1974.
63. Hockey, Robert V.: *Physical Fitness: The Pathway to Healthful Living,* 4th ed. St. Louis, Mosby, 1981.
64. Jankowski, L. W. and Evans, J. K.: The exercise capacity of blind children. *Journal of Visual Impairment and Blindness, 75(6):*248-251, June 1981.
65. Johnson, Leon and Londeree, Ben: *Motor Fitness Testing Manual for the Moderately Mentally Retarded.* Washington, D.C., AAHPER, 1982.
66. Joint Committee on Physical Fitness, Recreation, and Sports Medicine: Athletic activities by children with skeletal abnormalities. *Pediatrics, 51:*949-951, 1973.
67. Katz, Jane, with Bruning, Nancy P.: *Swimming for Total Fitness: A Progressive Aerobic Program.* Garden City, Doubleday, 1981.
68. Kelemen, Sue Jayne: *Fun With Aquatic Calisthenics,* Rev. ed. Lafayette, CA, Aquathenics of California, 1973.
69. Kisselle, Judy and Mazzeo, Karen S.: *Aerobic Dance: A Way to Fitness.* Englewood, Morton Pub., 1983.
70. Kuntzleman, Beth A. and the Editors of Consumer's Guide: *The Complete Guide to Aerobic Dancing,* New rev. ed. Skokie, IL, Publications International, 1982.
71. Larson, Leonard A. (Ed.): *Fitness, Health, and Work Capacity: International Standards for Assessment.* New York, MacMillan, 1974.
72. Laughlin, Sheila: A walking-jogging program for blind persons. *The New Outlook, 69(7):*312-313, September 1975.
73. Lawhorne, T. Wayne: Physical fitness for the mentally retarded: a reality. *Training School Bulletin, 62(2):*45-48, August 1966.
74. Lindsey, Dianne and O'Neal, Janet: Static and dynamic balance skills of eight year old deaf and hearing children. *American Annals of the Deaf, 121:*49-55, 1976.
75. Lundberg, Ake: Mechanical efficiency in bicycle ergometer work of young adults with cerebral palsy. *Developmental Medicine in Child Neurology, 17:*434-

439, 1975.

76. Lundberg, Ake, Ovenfors, Carl-Olof and Saltin, Beng: Effect of physical training on school-children with cerebral palsy. *Acta Paediatrica Scandinavica, 56*:182-188, 1967.

77. Marley, William P.: Asthma and exercise, a review. *Am Correc Ther J, 31(4)*:95-102, 1977.

78. Maryland State Board of Education: *Teacher's Helper: Physical Fitness for Handicapped Students.* Towson, 1983.

79. Mathews, Donald K.: *Measurement in Physical Education,* 5th ed. Philadelphia, Saunders, 1978.

80. Miller, Arthur G. and Sullivan, James V.: *Teaching Physical Activities to Impaired Youth: An Approach to Mainstreaming.* New York, Wiley, 1982.

81. Miller, David K. and Allen, T. Earl: *Fitness: A Lifetime Commitment,* 2nd ed. Minneapolis, Burgess, 1982.

82. Montessori, Maria: The Montessori Method, 5th ed. New York, Frederick A. Stokes, 1912.

83. Myers, Clayton R.: *The Official YMCA Physical Fitness Handbook.* New York, Popular Library, 1975.

84. Mykelbust, Helmer R.: Significance of etiology in motor performance of deaf children with special reference to meningitis. *American Journal of Psychology, 59*:249-258, 1946.

85. Neumann, Donald A.: Functional exercise position for treating persons with quadriplegia. *Physical Therapy, 60*:1291-1292, 1980.

86. Nunley, Rachel L.: A physical fitness program for the mentally retarded in the public schools. *Journal of the American Physical Therapy Association, 45*:946-954, 1965.

87. Oliver, James N.: The effect of physical conditioning exercises and activities on the mental characteristics of educationally sub-normal boys. *British Journal of Educational Psychology, 28(2)*:155-165, June 1958.

88. Pachalski, Adam and Mekarski, Tadeusz: Effect of swimming on increasing of cardio-respiratory capacity in paraplegics. *Paraplegia, 18(3)*:190-196, 1980.

89. Petersen, Kay H. and McElhenney, Thomas R.: Effects of a physical fitness program upon asthmatic boys. *Pediatrics, 35*:295-299, 1965.

90. Pollock, Douglas: Progressive resistive exercise device for quadriplegic patients. *Physical Therapy, 55*:992-993. 1975.

91. Pollock, Michael L., Wilmore, Jack H. and Fox, Samuel M. III: *Health and Fitness Through Physical Activity.* New York, Wiley, 1978.

92. Priest, Laurie: *Teach for Fitness: A Manual for Teaching Fitness Concepts in K-12 Physical Education.* Washington, D.C., ERIC Clearinghouse on Teacher Education, 1981.

93. Rarey, Kanute P. and Youtsey, John W.: *Respiratory Patient Care.* Englewood Cliffs, Prentice Hall, 1981.

94. Rarick, G. Lawrence, Widdop, James H. and Broadhead, Geoffrey D.: The physical fitness and motor performance of educable mentally retarded children. *Exceptional Children, 36*:509-519, 1970.

95. Reid, Elizabeth Lindsay and Morgan, Robert W.: Exercise prescription: a clinical trial. *Am J Public Health, 69*:591-595, 1979.

96. Robson, Peter: Cerebral palsy and physical fitness. *Developmental Medicine and Child Neurology, 14*:811-813, 1972.

97. Scherr, Merle S. and Frankel, Lawrence: Physical conditioning program for asthmatic children. *JAMA, 168*:1996-2000, 1958.

98. Seaman, Janet A. and DePauw, Karen R.: *The New Adapted Physical Education: A Developmental Approach.* Palo Alto, Mayfield, 1982.

99. Seguin, Edward: *Idiocy and its Treatment by the Physiological Method*, Reprint of 1866 edition. New York, Augustus M. Kelly, 1971.

100. Sengstock, Wayne L.: Physical fitness of mentally retarded boys. *Research Quarterly, 37(1)*:113-120, March 1966.

101. Sherrill, Claudine: *Adapted Physical Education and Recreation,* 2nd ed. Dubuque, Brown, 1981.

102. Solomon, Amiel and Pangle, Roy: Demonstrating physical fitness improvement in the EMR. *Exceptional Children, 34*:177-181, 1967.

103. Sorensen, Jacki with Bruns, Bill: *Aerobic Dancing.* New York, Rawson, Wade, 1979.

104. Stamford, Bryant A.: Cardiovascular endurance training for blind persons. *The New Outlook, 69(7)*:308-311, September 1975.

105. Stein, Julian U.: Physical fitness of mentally retarded boys relative to national age norms. *Rehabilitation Literature, 26(7)*:205-208, July 1965.

106. Stephens, Roberta: Running free: the use of a 'running cable' with blind adolescents who function on a retarded level. *The New Outlook, 67*:454-456, 1973.

107. Sullivan, Patricia E., Markos, Prudence D., and Minor, Mary Alice D.: *An Integrated Approach to Therapeutic Exercise: Theory and Clinical Application.* Reston, VA, Reston Pub. Co., 1982.

108. Van Dalen, Deobold B., and Bennett, Bruce L.: *A World History of Physical Education,* 2nd ed. Englewood Cliffs, NJ, Prentice Hall, 1971.

109. Vodola, Thomas M.:*A.C.T.I.V.E. Research Monograph: Competency-Based Teacher Training and Individualized-Personalized Physical Activity.* Oakhurst, NJ, Township of Ocean School District, 1978.

110. Weight training for wheelchair sports. *Practical Pointers, 2,* December 1978.

111. Weinberger, Miles: Exercise-induced asthma (editorial). *JAMA, 236*:447-448, 1975.

112. Wessel, Janet A.: *I Can: The Field Service Unit in Physical Education and Recreation for the Handicapped, Michigan State University.* Northbrook, IL, Hubbard, 1976.

113. Westcott, Wayne L.: *Strength Fitness: Physiological Principles and Training Techniques.* Boston, Allyn and Bacon, 1982.

114. Wheeler, Ruth Hook and Hooley, Agnes M.: *Physical Education for the Handicapped,* 2nd ed. Philadelphia, Lea & Febiger, 1976.

115. Wilmore, Jack H.: *Training for Sport and Activity* 2nd ed. Boston, Allyn and Bacon, 1982.

116. Wilson, Philip K., (Ed.): *Adult Fitness and Cardiac Rehabilitation.* Baltimore, University Park Press, 1975.

117. Winnick, Joseph P.: *Early Movement Experiences and Development: Habilitation and Remediation.* Philadelphia, Saunders, 1979.

118. Winnick, Joseph P. and Short, Francis X.: *The Physical Fitness of Sensory and Orthopedically Impaired Youth: Project UNIQUE, Final Report.* Brockport, NY, SUNY-Brockport, 1982.

119. Wiseman, Douglas C.: *A Practical Approach to Adapted Physical Education.* Reading, MA, Addison-Wesley, 1982.

120. Zwiren, Linda D. and Bar-Or, Oded: Responses to exercise of paraplegics who differ in conditioning level. *Medicine and Science in Sports, 7*:94-98, 1975.

PHOTO CREDITS

INDEX